HealThy Nurse

Escape Burnout &

Discover the Ultimate

Life / Work Balance

HealThy Nurse

Escape Burnout
&
Discover the Ultimate
Life / Work Balance

by Jennifer L. Carr, BSN, RN

Published by Matilda Publishing
Columbus, Indiana

Matilda Publishing
P.O. Box 1288
Columbus, Indiana 47202-1288
USA

www.healthynurse.com
info@healthynurse.com

ISBN, print edition: 0-9774909-0-4

ISBN, pdf edition: 0-9774909-1-2

Library of Congress Control Number: 2005938069

SAN 257-7208

Printed in the United States of America

Edited by Elyse K. Abraham, PhD

Stethoscope cover art by Susie Gregory
www.sadiespotsandpaintings.com

Cover by BookMasters, Inc.
www.bookmasters.com

Printed by BookMasters, Inc.
www.bookmasters.com

Dedication

For Granny –
a nurse, a writer, a visionary,
a dear friend, and a beautiful soul

Scholarship

One dollar from the sale of each book will go towards the *Norma Ludwick Memorial Nursing Scholarship.*

Acknowledgements

Endless thanks….

To my beautiful hero, James, my darling old soul, Tillie, and this miracle growing inside me – I love you truly, madly, and always!

To Jase – for believing in me when I didn't believe in myself.

To my parents – both here and in Oz – for always living and loving by example.

To my sisters – Boogs, Christy, Amanda, and Jenny – I love you!

Contents

The HealThy Nurse Transformation System™
- *Escape Burnout*
- *Discover the Ultimate Life / Work Balance*

Component II.
The *HealThy Nurse* Transformation Process™

The Core Concepts

1. Answer Your Own Call Light First

2. The Boomerang Principle

3. Expand Your Awareness (Optimal Awareness)

4. The Power of Choice

5. You Can't Change Others

6. The Law of Replacement

7. It Takes Courage to Live With Your Whole Soul

The Core strategies

1. Physualize (Beyond Visualization)

2. Take Time Out

3. Breathe

4. Walk

5. Let It Go

6. Activate

7. Meditate

Hope for the Future

Disclaimer

The author's best efforts were put forth in creating this book and making it as complete and accurate as possible. This publication and the information provided herein are current only up to the printing date. *HealThy Nurse* is meant to educate and entertain. It should be used only as a guide.

Neither the author nor Matilda Publishing shall assume responsibility or liability with respect to any injury or damage caused, or allegedly caused, either directly or indirectly, by the information contained in this book. The exercises and techniques presented in *HealThy Nurse* are not intended to replace the advice of your medical and/or psychiatric practitioner. You should discuss any concerns regarding individual limitations, conditions, or applicable modifications with your physician. You may return this book to the publisher for a complete and courteous refund if you do not wish to be bound by the above.

Introduction

"Healer, heal thyself." – Ancient Proverb

HealThy Nurse takes you through one nurse's journey – *my journey* – from burnout and despair to healing, happiness, and freedom. It is more than just a collection of memoirs or simply a commentary on the state of nursing today. *HealThy Nurse* promises radical honesty about what is really causing your burnout, about why you cope the way you do, and about how that coping is actually making you more miserable. More than that, it offers you the simple, yet powerful tools necessary to transform your life and take back your career.

Today's healthcare industry has become more about politics and money and less about the patient. As nurses, we find this deeply troubling. We see firsthand how patient satisfaction scores overshadow *real* patient care. The truth, which seems so painfully obvious to me, but which is overlooked or disregarded by the powers that be, is that satisfied nurses produce satisfied patients. Yet, nurses all over the world echo the same sentiments; we feel disillusioned, betrayed, de-valued, controlled, scripted – even *disposable.*

Once supportive and nurturing of one another, nurses now police each other out of fear. We feel as if our individuality has slowly been stripped away – but *I now know that this is because we've allowed it to be stripped away.* For all the nursing organizations, Web sites, and support groups devoted to nurses, I never understood why I felt so alone. Now I understand that many of us feel alone in a sea of millions, despite being part of the largest healthcare workforce in America. Overall, nurses are hurting, and our practice is struggling. Many of us feel tired, hope-less, and *burned-out.* This is the driving force behind a critical nursing shortage that is hovering on the verge of catastrophe.

Nursing is based in science. But it is also an art. My hope is for every nurse to recapture the artist within

The principles and strategies offered in **HealThy Nurse** *will challenge you. But they will also inspire you!*

As you embrace the very basic con-cepts and strategies that are part of the HealThy Nurse Trans-formation Process™, you will gradually, simply, and almost effortlessly transform your life.

herself[1] and to allow her uniqueness to shine through. We must quit following blindly, and just going through the motions because we're too tired, too beaten down, and too burned-out to do anything different.

With truth comes growth. As we work together through the HealThy Nurse Transformation System™, you will become more aware of your life and how you are responsible for creating it. You will begin to change it for the better. You will start *feeling* again. You will start thinking for yourself again (maybe for the first time ever). You will utilize those critical thinking and problem-solving skills and gut instincts that make you such a good caregiver. You will learn to trust those instincts again.

HealThy Nurse is not about blaming your burnout on the system, the powers that be, or anyone else. It is about taking personal responsibility for your own health and happiness. This is not always the most popular stance in today's world of talk shows and self-help books, which are quick to point a finger and seem to be blind to individual accountability. It is of no use bickering about why we are where we are or about how nursing and healthcare came to be such a distorted mess. Instead, it is of far greater value to look forward.

We must look to the future and get excited about where we can go from here.

The journey you are embarking on is a deeply spiritual one, without being specifically religious. It is a journey based in philosophy and psychology, and the principles and strategies provided are based on simple universal laws that are true for all of us.

Burnout can be difficult to put your finger on because it is intangible, and, as nurses, we tend to minimize our stress. It takes courage to recognize what we haven't been willing or able to see and to do something different. For all its wonders and accomplishments, Western medicine – *our* medicine – tends to medicate or mask symptoms rather than address and eliminate the root cause – "*Gallbladder bothering you? Let's take it out!*" "*Does your head ache? Pop this pill!*" As nurses, we very often do the same in "treating" ourselves. We slap a bandage on our stress and burnout by using any number of ineffective coping mechanisms. We self-medicate by using food, drink, bad relationships, or other unhealthy behaviors. While we may temporarily relieve the pain, we actually bring about more suffering, and we do nothing to address and eradicate the real cause.

The principles and strategies offered in *HealThy Nurse* will challenge you. But they will also inspire you. As you embrace the very basic concepts and strategies, you will gradually, simply, and almost effortlessly transform your life. Moreover, by beating your own burnout and living a healthy, happy life – living each day joyfully and with your whole soul – you will be leading by example. You will naturally lead and inspire others – at all levels – to do the same. You will then be doing your part to help optimize the role and function of nursing, greatly improving the care we give our patients, and helping us to become a truly powerful force – one nurse at a time.

Notes

[1]Sorry, guys. There is no gender-neutral pronoun.

Component I.
The Nurse Burnout Awareness Guide™

1

A Day in the Life

> "Idealism is what precedes experience;
> cynicism is what follows." – D. Wolf[1]

"F#@!% you, Nurse! You wait till I get one of them customer surveys!" These were some of the last words I heard from an ED patient under my care. The dialogue and scenario were hauntingly familiar. This particular "frequent flier" was well known in our department. I had just notified him that his request for a Demerol injection was denied by the attending ED physician. Just prior to that, the patient told me with a grin, *"It's the only thing that usually works,"* as he rated his chronic back pain at 10 out of 10 between sips of his Big Gulp® and yelling at Jerry Springer on the TV.

Sadly, I knew that this patient would probably receive a customer satisfaction survey in the mail, that he would actually take the time to fill it out (never mind that he couldn't spare ten seconds to throw on a condom before conceiving a fourth child he had no intention of supporting), that he would badmouth me, and that I might very likely find myself in my supervisor's office for a lecture about my bedside manner. And I knew, too, how that lecture would play out. I would stand there, defeated, knowing that there was little point in defending myself or recounting things as they had *actually* happened. After all, the customer is always right.

> At that moment, I knew that the system was broken and that it had broken me.
> I also knew that I couldn't fix it, and I couldn't take it any more. I did the only thing I could do to save myself, my family, and my sanity.
> I discovered a better way.

The scenario that day was not uncommon, and the shift was like any other. What was different was that I suddenly realized that everything I once loved about nursing was lost. And I was lost too.

It didn't start out this way. Patients had become customers, and they knew it. The sick ones were sicker. The ones who were not were more demanding and felt more entitled. (*Was I a nurse or a waitress?*) They were less respectful and less accountable. Nurse Managers had become suits, knee-deep in paperwork and politics, unsupportive, and far removed from the realities of what was actually happening on their units. The economics of healthcare, including compensating to cover the costs of treating the uninsured and underinsured, managed care and dwindling budgets now dictated our policies and practices, rather than the doctors who actually attended medical school and the nurses who actually nursed.

At that moment, I knew that the system was broken and that it had broken *me*. I also knew that I couldn't fix it, and I couldn't take it any more. I did the only thing I could do to save myself, my family, and my sanity. I discovered a better way.

This is my story.

Notes

[1]D. Wolf quotation from Mary Elizabeth Croft (2005), *How I Clobbered Every Bureaucratic Cash-Confiscatory Agency Known To Man: A Spiritual Economics Book on $$$ and Remembering Who You Are* (p. 12), an E-book available at http://www.wealth4freedom. com/law/Mary.htm

2

The Hard Facts

"The pure and simple truth is rarely pure
and never simple." – Oscar Wilde[1]

We've all read the headlines and heard about the nursing shortage on the evening news. We talk about it in our nurses' stations. More than that, we *feel* it. We know it's real because we are living it. The fact is that there is a critical and global shortage of nurses. According to Sigma Theta Tau International (2005), there are more than 11 million working nurses worldwide (p. 1). Yet, despite this seemingly large number, nursing organizations from 69 countries and every geographic area of the world report a nursing shortage, including the UK, Australia,

RIPPED FROM THE HEADLINES...

"Many Nurses Want Out!" (Detroit Free Press, 2001)

"Number of Nurses Shrinking despite Efforts to Retain Staff" (California Job Journal, 2002)

"Nurses around the World are Among the Least Satisfied Workers, and the Problem is Getting Worse" (AHRQ, 2001)

Canada, Germany, France, Switzerland, Poland, Denmark, The Netherlands, Zimbabwe, and Chile, just to name a few (International Council of Nurses, 2003, pp. 2-3).

Here in the United States, we are all too frequently reminded that patients and their families have lost trust in our hospitals. Today's nursing shortage is not just another cyclical shortage that can be solved with a few sign-on bonuses and a good recruitment campaign. The average age

> *We are facing a nursing shortage of tremendous proportions. It is driven not only by a diminished supply of new nurses entering the profession, but by a mass exodus of qualified nurses either abandoning their profession altogether or job-hopping as they search for happiness. This upheaval is a direct result of **burnout**.*

of today's RN is 40-something (American Nurses Association, 2001). The number of Americans age 65 and older is projected to grow from around 35 million today to more than 70 million by 2030 (Federal Interagency Forum on Aging-Related Statistics, 2004, p. 2). The inescapable conclusion is that as the aging nurse population nears retirement and the baby boomers enter their golden years, we will see fewer nurses in the workforce and more patients to care for. Not only are we in the

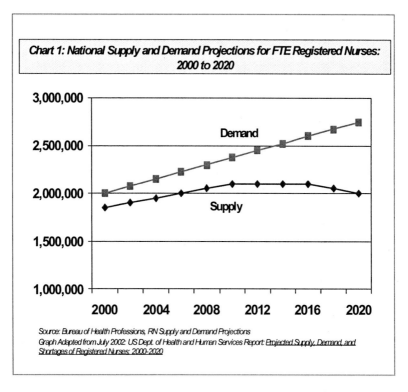

Chart 1: National Supply and Demand Projections for FTE Registered Nurses: 2000 to 2020

Source: Bureau of Health Professions, RN Supply and Demand Projections
Graph Adapted from July 2002: US Dept. of Health and Human Services Report: Projected Supply, Demand, and Shortages of Registered Nurses: 2000-2020

midst of a nursing shortage, but we are facing a nursing shortage of *tremendous proportions.*

This nursing shortage is driven not only by a diminished supply of new nurses entering the profession, but by a mass exodus of qualified nurses either abandoning their profession altogether or job-hopping as they search for happiness. **This upheaval in the healthcare industry is a direct result of burnout.**

The hard truth is that, by 2010, the number of nurses needed will vastly outstrip the number available.

Looking into the not so distant future, the Federal Bureau of Health Professions reported in July 2002 that the demand for RNs is expected to grow from 2 million to 2.8 million by 2020 (see Chart 1 above). This growth will result in a 29 percent shortage, up from 6 percent in 2000 (p. 2). If that doesn't scare people, it should. **We are on the verge of a potential catastrophe in healthcare.**

According to the American Nurses Association (2005), there are nearly 3 million Registered Nurses in the United States. We are the largest healthcare workforce in America and the lifeblood of the medical community. And in fact, Gallup poles have consistently shown that the public perceives nurses to be among the most trustworthy, capable, and conscientious caregivers. However, even though there are more than enough nurses to fill the void, hospitals are having a hard time finding enough nurses to work under current conditions. **Despite caring for sicker patients, nurses have fewer resources and bigger workloads.**

Unfortunately, those in specialty areas are often the hardest hit. Experienced nurses are increasingly hard to come by. The International Council of Nurses reported in 2003 the following alarming statistic concerning the ratio of experienced nurses to new graduates (p. 4).

- 1990: 90% experienced nurses to 10% new graduates.
- 2000: 50% experienced nurses to 50% new graduates.

We all know why this is dangerous on so many levels. Not only is it absolutely frightening for our patients, but it puts more stress on those of us experienced nurses who are increasingly among the struggling minority.

Extensive research has shown that the nursing shortage has a very direct impact on the quality of patient care and outcomes. The International Council of Nurses (2003) reported that *"for each additional year of nursing experience present in the clinical unit of an urban hospital, six fewer patients died of every 1,000 discharged"* (p. 4). **The bottom line is that when experienced nurses burn out and walk away, more patients die.**

A national online survey by the American Nurses Association released in February 2001 revealed some startling statistics about how nurses view their profession and current conditions.

- An alarming 41.5% *"would NOT feel confident having someone close to them receive care in the facility in which they work"* (p. 11).
- 20% indicated that they were *"frightened for their patients"* (p. 9).
- Over half (54.8%) *"would not recommend the nursing profession to their children or friends"* (p. 12).

In 2002, the Journal of the American Medical Association (JAMA) reported the following disturbing statistics:

> The shortage of hospital nurses may be linked to unrealistic nurse workloads. Forty percent of hospital nurses have burnout levels that exceed the norms for healthcare workers. Job dissatisfaction among hospital nurses is 4 times greater than the average for all US workers, and 1 in 5 hospital nurses report that they intend to leave their current job within a year. (Aiken, Clarke, Sloane, Sochalski, & Silber, 2002, p. 1987)

As nurses, we *see* firsthand how the nursing shortage is eroding patient care. This demanding and oppressive environment is chasing nurses away, forcing them to leave out of pain and frustration. Many nurses are so disenchanted that they are choosing not to use their degrees at all. **The truth is that we are overwhelmed**

and stuck in a vicious cycle, with stress at its core and burnout the painful end result.

The government, hospitals, and even the media have answered the nursing shortage crisis by launching aggressive recruitment campaigns and introducing legislation to fund nursing programs. Nursing organizations are providing scholarships and loan repayment incentives, and are taking on innovative recruitment techniques. However, these efforts do little to address the real problem – *burnout*.

> *The truth is that we are overwhelmed and we are stuck in a vicious cycle, with stress at its core and burnout the painful end result.*

It is all well and good to get prospective nurses into what can be – or once was – such a rewarding and meaningful career, but it is of absolutely no use if we do not face and address the core issues that are driving our nurses away. In her book, *Where Have All The Nurses Gone? The Impact Of The Nursing Shortage On American Healthcare*, Faye Satterly, RN examined the nursing shortage. She says of nurses today:

They are tired, they feel unappreciated and unheard, and they worry about the level of responsibility falling on their shoulders. It is easy to dismiss them as complainers, but it would be more accurate to see them as depressed, 'burned out'. And it is important that we understand why, because it is their feelings of hopelessness and being overwhelmed that are driving the nursing shortage. (p. 40)

Additionally, discussing the nurses who responded to The ANA Staffing Survey as well as to her own survey, Satterly says that they

expressed a surprising amount of emotion. They felt betrayed. They had lost faith in their institutions and distrusted the motivations of those who manage the healthcare facilities. They still felt loyal to the patients and the mission of their profession, but they no longer believed in their employers' mission. (p. 79)

What about Retention?

Jeanna Bozell, RN, founder of NurseQuest, summed up the retention situation accurately when she said,

You can recruit till the cows come home, and that's what we see nurse recruiters in hospitals doing. Pull out all the stops, do the sign-on bonuses, basically bribe them in some way to get them in the door. But until you can stop the bleeding, they're coming in the front door and leaving out the back door. (*NurseWeek*, 2004, p. 4)

In a time when nurses are overwhelmed with customer satisfaction surveys and hospital politics in a healthcare system that is hanging on by a thread, what can we offer those who have already given their hearts and souls and who are wondering how much longer they can hold on? Nurses need a lifeline to save them from the vicious cycle of burnout. They need hope and real-life powerful tools to help them alleviate stress and gain more energy, health, happiness, and balance.

The bottom line is that we are all responsible for our own happiness. There are things you can do *right now* to change how you look at the world and your place in it – today and for the rest of your life. Nursing will always be hard work, but you *can* make burnout a thing of the past. Not only will you be helping yourself, you'll be doing your part to save and transform our sick healthcare industry. **Because the only way nursing can be saved is one nurse at a time.**

Notes

[1]Oscar Wilde quote from *The Importance of Being Ernest* (1895), retrieved October 5, 2005 from http://www.quotationspage.com/quote/3808.html

References

Agency for Healthcare Research and Quality (AHRQ). (2001, August). *Nursing Research: Nurses around the world are among the least satisfied workers, and the problem is getting worse. Research Activities, No. 252* (p. 1). United States Dept. of Health and Human Services. Retrieved July 25, 2005 from http://www.ahrq.gov/re search/aug01/801RA12.htm

Aiken, L. H., Clarke, S. P., Sloane, D. M., Sochalski, J., & Silber, J. H. (2002). Hospital nurse staffing and patient mortality, nurse burnout, and job dissatisfaction [Electronic Version]. *JAMA, Journal of the American Medical Association, 288*(16), 1987-1993. Retrieved July 28, 2005, from www.jama.com

American Nurses Association (ANA). (2005). About the American Nurses Association. Retrieved September 1, 2005 from http://nursingworld.org/ about/

American Nurses Association (ANA). (2001, February 6). Analysis of American Nurses Association staffing survey. Retrieved July 25, 2005 from http://www.nursingworld.org/staffing/ana_pdf.pdf

Federal Interagency Forum on Aging-Related Statistics. (2004). Older Americans 2004: Key Indicators of Well-Being. Retrieved July 25, 2005 from http://www.agingstats.gov/chartbook2004/population.html

Griffin, Cynthia E. (2002, May 19). Number of nurses shrinking despite efforts to retain staff. *California Job Journal* (p. 1). Retrieved August 28, 2005 from http://www.jobjournal.com/article_printer.asp?artid=507

International Council of Nurses. (2003, January - March). Global issues in the supply and demand of nurses. *Socio-Economic News, SEW News.* Retrieved July 25, 2005 from http://www.icn.ch/sewjan-march03.htm

Kennedy, Sheryl. (2001, April 20). Many nurses want out. *Detroit Free Press* (p. 1). Retrieved August 28, 2005 from http://www.freep.com/money/business/nurse20_20010420.htm

McPeck, Phil. (2004, February 23). Can we fix it? Nursing experts say underlying changes in the image and working conditions of RNs are critical to addressing the shortage. *NurseWeek News.* Retrieved July 18, 2005 from http://www.nursew eek.com/news/features/042/shortage_print.html

Satterly, Faye. (2004). *Where Have All The Nurses Gone? The Impact Of The Nursing Shortage On American Healthcare.* Amherst, NY: Prometheus Books.

Sigma Theta Tau International Honor Society of Nurses. (2005). Benefits of nurses as sources. Retrieved July 28, 2005 from http://www.nursing society.org/media/benefitsofnurses_sources. html

US Department of Health and Human Services, Health Resources and Services Administration, Bureau of Health Professions, National Center For Health Workforce Analysis. (2002). *Projected Supply, Demand, and Shortages of Registered Nurses: 2000-2020.* Retrieved July 28, 2005 from ftw://ftp.hrsa.gov/bhpr/nationalcenter/rnpro ject.pdf

3

Always On Call

"Wisdom begins in wonder."
— Socrates[1] (469-399 BC)

Being a nurse is not just a job. **It is who we are.**
We are caregivers. By nature, we tend to be pleasers,
and we have a need to nurture others. But let's face it,
along with the altruism can come a bit of a martyr complex. Unfortunately, the very thing that makes us good
nurses — caring for others and putting them first — is often what makes us so unhappy, unhealthy, over-
stressed, and in need of healing ourselves.

Nursing is a job we take with us wherever we go.
We are "always on call" — whether it's a sick family
member, a neighbor with an *"I hate to bother you with
this, but–"* medical question, or an ankle injury at our
kid's soccer game. Most of us have busy lives and
families to care for after a long day (or night) on the job.
It seems never ending.

The old adage *you can't take care of others until
you take care of yourself first* is so true. But alas, like

many things in life, it is easier said than done. Many of us become lost in the day-to-day activities of life, not stopping to think about what we're really doing, if it's working for us, or even if it's what we really want – until something happens and we suddenly discover that we've lost ourselves. I know I did.

I've never been "Nancy Nurse," believe me. But I loved being a nurse, and I was good at it. However, after 10 years in an Emergency Department, I had become so over-stressed, exhausted, and utterly paralyzed with fear and burnout that I didn't know who I was anymore, or what was beyond those ED doors. I may have been the "go to girl" when nobody could get a line, but I wasn't nearly the nurse I could have been if I had known then what I know now. I have learned that it doesn't matter how strong our skills are, or how much experience we have, or how many letters we have behind our name, if our soul is sick. After what I now lovingly refer to as "my meltdown" (more about that to follow), many tears, and a lot of heavy-duty soul searching, I began to "see the light" so to speak. And what a beautiful light it is.

I am a nurse, yes. But that's not all I am. I am a wife, a mother, a daughter, a sister, a friend, a woman, a person…. I finally realized that the rest of my life was suffering, because my job had made me so miserable (or rather, because I had *allowed* it to make me so miserable). I knew I was "stressed-out," but I had no idea how deep it ran or how it was affecting every area of my life. Once I got a handle on that and made the very conscious **choice** to create a lifestyle that relieves stress on a daily basis and to care for and feed my body, mind, and soul, I became someone else. Someone so much better. Someone much happier. Someone free. Someone I love dearly. Someone I love being.

Our work has always been hard, even exhausting. But most of us can remember a time when we had fun and even laughed. When we were not so burned-out that we could barely see past our own stress and drama. A time when we looked out for each other. When we left our shift feeling fulfilled, empowered, and maybe even looking forward to the next one, rather than feeling depleted, empty, and hopeless. As nurses, we will always see death, despair, and the ugliness of life, but we **can** turn the ship around and look toward a happier future.

Notes

[1]Socrates quote retrieved July 25, 2005 from http://www.brainyquote.com/quotes/quotes/s/socrates1 01211.html

4

My Story

"I was one of those breathing tornadoes.
But now I live at the eye of the storm."
– Ben Lee[1] (Australian Songwriter)

I used to love being a nurse. Or perhaps it was the *idea* of nursing and what it once meant to me. After several years at Indiana University studying everything from art to journalism to psychology, I finally settled on a career in nursing. Since I come from a long line of nurses and doctors, that seemed like a natural choice. I earned a Bachelor of Science in Nursing in 1994. My first job was in an ICU at a Level One Trauma Center in Indianapolis, Indiana. Having worked as a Student Extern on the unit during my last year of school, I knew that I was very fortunate to get the job, as most new grads have to "pay their dues" before being allowed to work in a critical care arena. I loved it.

The Emergency Department followed a brief stint in Australia with the beautiful man who would become my husband. We returned to my hometown to tie the knot, and I happily took a job in our local hospital. I was proud to work along side my father, a physician and 30-year ED veteran – who also happens to be as good as they get. The excitement, diversity, and grittiness of the ED suited me.

Sadly though, somewhere along the line, I went from wanting to save the world to *"Why can't you miserable ingrates go get a J-O-B?!?!"* I saw my friends and colleagues walk away, one by one, beaten and burned-out. I commiserated with them, and I tried, halfheartedly, to convince them to stick with it. All the while, I failed to recognize my own downward spiral towards burnout.

While nursing can be immensely fulfilling and rewarding, it is also a job unlike any other. We see a side of life – and death – that most people only catch a glimpse of. It is easy to feel as if no one really understands the ugliness and intense stress that we can face with each and every shift. It's not as if we get called into the principle's office if we miss a deadline. If we make an error, someone could die. Add to that a critical nursing shortage, weekends and holidays away from our families, not having a moment to breathe along the way, and not having the tools to cope, and it is no surprise that we're headed for disaster.

Eventually, I became so miserable that I spent every moment off duty dreading the next shift and counting the days until I had to go back. I regretfully confess that I was hell to live with. I was so busy dreading work, complaining about work, and just generally feeling sorry for myself that I hardly had time *to be in the moment* and to enjoy my husband and daughter, both of whom I love fiercely. Although I have a wonderfully supportive husband and never once felt as if my marriage was in jeopardy, it is easy to see why the divorce rate is so high among nurses and those in the medical profession. Between the bad hours, an intensely stressful job, and the unhealthy habits that often accompany the job, many marriages and relationships suffer.

Work had become so miserable that I couldn't wait to get home and "unwind" with a beer (or three) and chain-smoke until my lungs hurt. I went from someone who loved the gym to a sluggish blob of self-pity who turned to emotional eating to numb the pain. I cried – a lot. I remember catching a glimpse of myself in a mirror and being shocked at the reflection staring back at me. *Who's fat ass was that?* Like the proverbial ED patient staring in shock at the x-ray clearly portraying the cucumber he'd shoved up his rectum and asking incredulously *"How'd that get there?!"*, I wondered how I'd reached such a state. I realized that my burnout was more than a change in departments or even hospitals could fix.

My friends and family knew I was unhappy at work. I remember telling them (not intending all the drama it now seems to imply) *"That place is rotting my soul."* I felt absolutely paralyzed, desperately wanting to get out and do something else, but unable to make the move.

Judy, my friend, neighbor, and, incidentally, one of the best bakers I know, calls herself an "ex-nurse" after suffering her own burnout many years ago and walking away from the profession entirely. Without knowing it, she impacted my life tremendously with one sentence on a fateful cold November afternoon. She said, *"Jen, whatever you do, don't live your life in fear like I did."* Those words echoed in my heart and mind over the next days and months. They still do.

I am so blessed in my life to have been born of a long line of strong women – matriarchs in the truest sense of the word. My mother's side of the family has always been what some might call "forward-thinking" – perhaps too much so for some people. My relatives were "hippies" long before hippies were cool. One of the most influential and important people in my life has been my grandmother, Norma Ludwick. Granny was a nurse, a writer, a visionary, and always ahead of her time. She truly was my kindred spirit. In a way, she was the one who lead me to this project.

Although I could never do Granny justice, she was a wildly funny woman who loved life and was open to all its possibilities. She wore outlandish clothes and would let us style her hair however we wanted – proudly wearing her silver cornrows to the theatre with careless disregard for what anyone else might think. She always managed to find humor in things and could muster something positive from even the darkest of situations. She never took herself too seriously and seemed to embrace each moment with all she had. She was kind beyond words. She understood the true joy of giving and did it without motivation. When in her presence, I knew without doubt that I was loved wildly and unconditionally. Quite simply, Granny "got it."

Sadly, I lost her when I was sixteen. She was far too young to go, and I miss her every day. But I know that she is with me, and I feel her all around me. Thankfully, my mother *is* my grandmother in so many ways. Hopefully, I am too. I have learned to have no regrets in my life. I do, however, wish that I could have known my grandmother as a fellow woman, rather than as the young girl who could see her for little more than the fabulously fun Granny that she was.

Fortunately, Granny left behind countless journals. She wrote endlessly about her journey through life and her path towards self-discovery, true happiness, and the real meaning of life (with a few "wafer thin mints" thrown in for good measure – Granny was a huge Monty Python fan).

Through her journals, I learned that Granny was not as I had idealized her, but even better. Along with her wisdom and insights, she had insecurities and heartaches. She was searching and struggling just like the rest of us. I discovered that she was an avid student of what she referred to as "the perennial tradition" – the universal integration of psychology, philosophy, and spirituality as it relates to personal growth and evolution. She read books and took part in discussion groups about self-discovery long before it was in vogue. As an adult, I poured over her journals in an attempt to reconnect and to get to know her again. Sometimes, I felt as if I were reading my own journals. I read the books she had read, and I studied her notes. Over the years, I absorbed so much without even realizing it. Looking back, it probably influenced my decision to become a nurse – as well as my decision to become a writer.

When I was feeling lost in my life and struggling with burnout, I revisited those journals and reread some of those books. I started to think about how I might take some of those age-old principles and apply them to the hectic world of nursing. Could it work? Perhaps it was divine intervention, perhaps it was Granny, or perhaps it was just time. I formulated a plan. I developed seven basic principles and seven basic strategies that I thought would work for nurses struggling with burnout. Over the next six months, I quietly practiced the principles and strategies that I had developed. I was sure my workmates would think I was crazy if I let them in on my little secret.

The concepts were so simple and so basic, yet they worked! Over time, I took notes and tweaked the principles and strategies. Before I knew it, I was a different person. It dawned on me that my life was mine again and that I was no longer a stressed out, burned-out mess at work or at home. My future changed in that instant.

I knew that I needed to share what I had learned with other nurses, but I was terrified to leave my comfort zone – as uncomfortable as it had become. I made the decision to be true to myself and to follow my gut. (Trusting our instincts is one of the most important tools we have as nurses. How could I have lost that?) Something finally clicked, and the floodgates opened. I made the first real choice I had made in a long time. I turned in my resignation the very next day, and I embarked on this wonderful journey. I became determined to share what I had learned and to coach others towards a healthy and happy nursing career.

Notes

[1]Ben Lee quote from the song "Into the Dark," written and performed by Ben Lee on the album *Awake is the New Sleep* (2005), New West Records, LLC, 9215 Olympic Blvd., Los Angeles, CA 90212, www.newwest records.com and www.ben-lee.com

5

The Nurse's Dilemma

"Without stress, there would be no life."
– Hans Selye[1] (Canadian physiologist)

No, you're not going crazy. And yes, your job is becoming more difficult. The nursing shortage is hotly debated today, and the solution is complex and daunting at best. The cause, however, can be traced to one thing – **burnout**. This may seem overly simplistic, but nurse burnout is part of a vicious cycle that so many of us are caught in.

The growing nursing shortage and burnout are deeply interrelated, which makes eliminating them even more difficult. The nursing shortage is made worse by increased burnout, which generates a dramatic increase in workload for

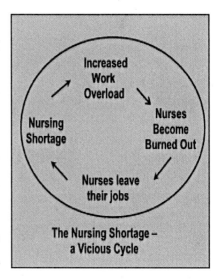

Increased Work Overload

Nurses Become Burned Out

Nursing Shortage

Nurses leave their jobs

The Nursing Shortage – a Vicious Cycle

those nurses who are left behind. The increase in workload, in turn, leads to more burn out, which, of course, increases the nursing shortage, and so on, and so on. It is the proverbial unending vicious cycle. Unfortunately, we are so busy trying to catch up that we hardly have time to recognize what's happening to us, let alone thwart the attack.

The Link between Chronic *Stress* & Disease

Chronic stress leads to physical and psychological ailments that affect virtually every system in the human body. Here are a few. Any of them ring a bell?

- *depression*
- *anxiety disorders, such as panic attacks, phobias, and obsessive compulsive fears*
- *weight gain, weight loss, or eating disorders*
- *sleep disturbance*
- *cancer*
- *cardiovascular problems, such as heart disease, stroke, chest pain, hypertension, increased heart rate, and shortness of breath*
- *sexual and reproductive dysfunction*
- *addiction, including self-medication and unhealthy lifestyle*
- *allergies*
- *increased susceptibility to infection and immune disorders*
- *diabetes*
- *migraine and tension headaches*
- *gastrointestinal problems, such as inflammatory bowel disease, irritable bowel syndrome and peptic ulcers*

Nursing can be quite stressful under optimum conditions. (Let's face it – some of us are drawn to the profession to feed the adrenaline junkie lurking within us.) As nurses, we must remain calm under pressure and work through anything. But just because we get the right meds to the right patients at the right time or work well in a code and are "good under pressure," does not mean our bodies and minds are not feeling the effects of stress.

What is Stress?

Stress is such a common part of our lives that it might be surprising to learn that the term as we know it was introduced just over fifty years ago. Hans Selye, a Canadian physiologist, is considered to be the "Father of Stress." In 1950, Selye first coined the term *stress* as it is used today in his book *The Physiology and Pathology of Exposure to Stress.*

Selye's research revealed that there are two kinds of stress – *Eustress* and *Distress.* Eustress is positive stress. It is necessary to keep us functioning, and adds a bit of spice to life. Distress is negative stress and is created when our system has become overloaded (Selye, 1978).

Over the years, stress has been studied extensively, and millions of books promising ways to beat it have been published. Yet, problems resulting from stress are more pervasive in our culture today than ever before.

The Truth about Stress

Stress evokes a fight or flight response within us. Our minds signal our bodies to gear up for the potential threat, and our response can be likened to that of a jet airplane readying for take-off. Of course, not all stress is bad. The stress that is generated as a result of exciting or challenging events, such as a code or the birth of a child, is necessary and actually serves to enhance our performance. In fact, life would be boring without a bit of stress.

> "Stress, in addition to being itself, was also the cause of itself, and the result of itself."
> – Hans Selye (cited in Rosch)

Chronic stress, however, is another issue entirely. Imagine a jet airplane constantly in take-off mode. Obviously, the engine would eventually *burn out*. Likewise, when the body is kept in a constant state of stress or "fight mode," fatigue and damage ultimately result. If we don't allow time for rest and repair, our bodies become seriously compromised. As a result, the risk of injury and illness escalates. This chronic over-stimulation of the autonomic nervous system, without rest, creates the stress that ends up killing us in a variety of ways. It is no wonder that stress has been called the world's number one killer.

Search the Web and you will find over 250,000 sites dedicated to stress and the ailments it can cause. Emotional stress has very real physical implications. For instance, the American Psychological Association (APA) (2005, pp. 1-2) reports that:

- *Between 75 and 90 percent of all physician office visits are for stress-related ailments and complaints.*

- *Stress is linked to the six leading causes of death – heart disease, cancer, lung ailments, accidents, cirrhosis of the liver, and suicide.*

Moreover, chronic stress leads to a broad spectrum of physical and psychological ailments, affecting virtually *every* body system.

Stress is not just expensive emotionally and physically, but fiscally as well. According to the APA

(2005), "Workplace stress causes approximately one million US employees to miss work each day" (p. 3). For our purposes, it is also significant to note that a number of studies have shown that there is a correlation between workplace stress and nurses' morale, job satisfaction, commitment to the organization, and intent to quit (Rosenstein, 2002). **Nurses are caring for sicker patients with fewer resources, and most of us don't know how to cope with stress in a healthy manner.**

When we do not relieve stress on a daily basis, it builds. We become overloaded with stress, and we essentially "store" the stress demands until we have time to catch up. Consider an analogy posed by Dr. Selye.[2] Imagine an office worker with stacks and stacks of paperwork piling up on her desk. If she doesn't deal with them, or "catch up," the stacks of paperwork create problems as they continue to grow, and they will prevent her from working at her full capacity. How many of us have awakened in the middle of the night in a panic, asking ourselves, *"Did I give that med?"* How many of us find ourselves lying awake at night, unable to fall asleep to the backdrop of monitor alarms echoing in our minds?

What really causes Stress?

We have been conditioned to accept that our family's medical history greatly determines our future health. Their cancers will become our cancers. Their biological weaknesses will become ours. We are helpless against inherited diseases. But what if the real culprit is *stress* rather than genetics?

As is often the case in life, the *perceived* problem is not always the *real* problem. We tend to view stress as an outside threat or invader – something "out there." But the reality is that stress is not an external thing. What may be stressful to one individual may not trigger stress in another. What affects one person may have no effect on another.

In reality, it is our beliefs – what we believe about ourselves and our world – that form our perceptions. Our perceptions are the pictures or stories that we accept as the truth or reality of our lives (more on this later). Your perceptions, pictures, or stories – whatever you want to call them – trigger your reactions to your environment. So then, when we discover that **we have the power to change our beliefs or pictures**, stress is no longer a threat waiting "out there." Through visualization (physualization), replacement,

Are You Trapped in the Nurses Dilemma?

Burnout has some very definite characteristics. Here are a few warning signs:

- *feeling exhausted and physically overloaded*
- *feeling psychologically and emotionally overwhelmed*
- *crying before, during, or after a shift*
- *lack of energy and vitality for life*
- *frustration and anxiety*
- *an alarming absence of life / work balance*
- *the nagging feeling that you are taking care of everyone (patients, friends, family, etc.) but yourself*
- *emotional eating & drinking to numb the pain of work*
- *weight gain or weight loss*

and expanding our awareness, we can replace our old pictures and stories with positive healthy ones that empower and free us. Ultimately, we *can* greatly reduce stress and thus, eliminate burnout from our lives.

How Stress is related to Burnout

Anyone can experience burnout. In order to burn out, one must be alight to begin with. This means that burnout can only happen to those of us who are passionate about our work. Nurses are particularly at risk for burnout because we are so deeply committed to our field, and in fact, many of us derive our own sense of identity from our work. We energetically begin our careers with great aspirations to help others and to make a difference in the lives of our patients. But unfortunately, our selflessness can lead to really *losing ourselves*.

In addition, we tend to minimize our stress and put self-care on the back burner. Ultimately, the line between work and personal life becomes blurred. Over time, I have come to realize what experts in the field of integrated / holistic healing practices have known for centuries – the body, mind, and soul are interrelated and cannot be considered separate entities. **We must care for our *whole* self in order to live with our whole soul.** And we cannot care for others unless we first care for ourselves.

Although nursing can be exciting and rewarding, it can also be emotionally charged and stressful. As nurses, we all share certain characteristics, but our personalities vary widely. Personalities that we might otherwise find endearing can clash with our own when tension is high and burnout is lurking. Additionally, our patients also provide a vast array of personalities, cultures, and lifestyles (thank goodness! this is one of my favorite aspects of nursing), which further increases the potential for stress and drama during tense situations. Along with this, we are challenged with a nursing shortage out of control, physical and emotional exhaustion, exposure to disease, injury and assault, and an increasing sense of disillusionment. It is not surprising that we find ourselves on the road to *burnout.*

The Road to Nurse Burnout

When we experience constant work overload, we are over-stressing our mind and body systems. This eventually leads to our mind and body systems becoming overwhelmed and beginning to break down, which leads to emotional coping and reactivity. Our energy becomes depleted and our resistance low, leaving us susceptible to exhaustion, frustration, depression, and illness.

All this constant and increasing anxiety and stress on our mind and body eventually leads to a broken spirit and disillusionment, with the end result being burnout. Although we may experience a subtle awareness of burnout, we tend to ignore it because it becomes such a familiar, almost comfortable, part of our lives.

The Road to Nurse Burnout

How does a nurse go from healthy, happy, and alight with passion about her work to *burned out*? The process goes like this:

The nurse copes with constant work overload.

⇩

Her mind / body systems become over-stressed.

⇩

Her overwhelmed mind / body systems begin to breakdown.

⇩

She resorts to emotional coping and reactivity to deal with the stress.

⇩

She experiences low energy and a low resistance to disease.

⇩

She experiences total exhaustion, detachment, and a broken spirit.

⇩

Burnout

Understanding Nurse Burnout

The road to nurse burnout is complex. Let's look more closely at the process that occurs as a nurse burns out.

1. **Constant Work Overload** – With the nursing shortage driving work overload, nurses are collectively on the verge of a mass break-down. We are forced to work beyond our normal physical capacity. Startling nurse-patient ratios, mandatory overtime (either overtly stated or implied, *"If you don't work these extra shifts, you're not a team player"*), more demands with fewer resources, brutal schedules with few (if any) breaks, and little support from management cause work over-load, which leads to over-stressed mind / body systems.

2. **Mind / Body Systems become Over-Stressed** – Remember, our body, mind, and spirit are not independent entities. One *abso-lutely* affects the other. When we continually over-stress our mind and body without taking

time to release that stress and feed our spirit, we begin our journey towards the next step – our mind / body systems become overwhelmed by the constant overload and begin to break down.

3. *Overwhelmed Mind / Body Systems begin to Break Down* – This step is recognized by excessive crying, fear, anxiety, depression, and sadness. We may experience these symptoms more and more frequently. Family life or personal relationships may become strained.

4. *Emotional Coping and Reactivity* – When we do not have the tools to release stress and refresh ourselves effectively, the daily choices we make to cope are almost always going to wear us down and propel us further down the road to burnout – and further away from a healthy, energetic, and balanced life. We numb ourselves with food, smoking, drinking, excessive TV *("I'd rather watch someone else's life rather than face my own"*

or *"At least I'm not **that** poor slob"),* drugs, or whatever the escape of choice is. We may become increasingly detached. We may depersonalize, treating our patients and co-workers in a callous or uncaring manner. These ineffective coping mechanisms make things worse and lead us closer to burnout.

5. ***Low Energy and Low Resistance to Disease*** – Ineffective coping mechanisms and an unhealthy lifestyle ultimately lead to even less energy and decreased resistance to disease. We become more susceptible to any number of physical and emotional ailments. As our threshold lowers, almost everyone and everything annoys us. We may continue to withdraw from the outside world as a means of self-preservation (however misguided that choice may be). We may experience weight gain or weight loss, escalating anxiety disorders, and deepening depression. We are often sick, and absenteeism may increase. We can feel burnout settling in and making itself comfortable.

6. **Exhaustion, Detachment, and a Broken Spirit** – The last step is physical, emotional, and spiritual exhaustion. We become completely withdrawn and cynical. We feel spent and empty. We no longer derive any satisfaction from our work, and we no longer want to do it. We may sabotage or even walk away from our personal relationships. Crying all the time may evolve into an eerie inability to cry. Sleeplessness may transform into sleeping all the time. Whatever ineffective coping mechanisms we use escalate, and we become even more miserable. We are physically and emotionally exhausted. We have arrived in our own personal hell. This is **burnout**. Feeling hopeless and disillusioned, we might shift to a position far removed from patient care or leave nursing all together.

The road to burnout and the end result are essentially the same and equally painful for every nurse, but some nurses arrive at burnout much faster than others. For some of us, the road to burnout is a short one that ends abruptly – as when new nurses with bright futures, barely out of school, quickly abandon the profession when their job fails to live up to their expectations. Most of us go into nursing with the expectation that we will provide patient care, use our critical thinking skills, and play an important role as a professional rather than be just

"I am personally finding the stress level of new grads working in our critical care environment a big issue. They are easily burned out and eaten up by our older, burned-out staff. The workload is so intense. We can't get experienced help and we can't keep good help. It's a vicious cycle."
– Arlene Watrobski,[3] BSN, RN, CEN, CCRN, Patient Care Coordinator, Emergency Department, Active Critical Care Nurse for 35 years

another disposable number. So, it is not surprising that many new nurses quickly become disillusioned as they realize that today's nurse is overwhelmed with non-nursing tasks, unrealistic workloads and politics. This, combined with poor working conditions and lack of support from fellow nurses and management (many of whom are cynical and on the road to burnout themselves), makes for a quick trip down the road to burnout.

Alternatively, for some of us, the road can be a long and winding one, with several stops along the way in the form of temporary leaves of absence, chronic (often preventable) illness, and shuffling positions in a half-hearted attempt to refresh and rejuvenate our careers. We all know nurses who have been struggling with the nurse's dilemma too long without putting self-care first. They have been on the road to burnout for some time and either fail to recognize it or are unwilling to give up the fight. Although they may be admired for their dedication, they ultimately bring down morale and hamper everyone else's productivity and ability to do their job. And truth be told, they aren't doing their patients, co-workers, or, more importantly, *themselves* any favors by sticking around – unless they take a right turn and begin to *HealThy Nurse*. The good news is that, no matter how long the road to burnout is or at which point each nurse finds herself, there is always hope.

Burnout is a potential threat facing every nurse. The reality is that to practice nursing today, many nurses must cope with deplorable working conditions and risk burnout, or they must leave

The Nurse's Dilemma

The Nurse's Dilemma is the dark side of nursing that we must acknowledge. A great many nurses must face the nurse's dilemma every day. They must choose either to work under deplorable working conditions, or to leave their nursing careers.

the nursing profession. For nurses who truly love nursing, as I do, this is an impossible choice. This is the *Nurse's Dilemma*. Increasing numbers of nurses must face the nurse's dilemma every day.

The vicious nursing shortage cycle continues as more nurses leave, frustrated and burned out. The remaining nurses are left with an even bigger workload, which causes more burnout, which results in more nurses leaving, which increases the nursing shortage, which increases the workload of those nurses left behind, and so on. On an individual scale, the Nurse's Dilemma becomes harder to manage as work becomes more overwhelming and physical and emotional energy continue to dwindle. Ultimately, the nurse finds herself at the end of the road, burned out and ready to give up the fight. The cycle continues.

Burnout is difficult to eliminate because it is both the cause and the effect of the nursing shortage. Our healthcare industry is sick and major changes are needed in order to save it. However, before we can begin to tackle the much broader challenge of the nursing shortage, we must each save ourselves first.

It has long been said that we cannot correct a problem until we first acknowledge that it exists. Now that you are more consciously aware of what is happening, you can identify the signs and symptoms of burnout, diagnose the problem, and you can begin to heal yourself. You can prevent burnout from creeping back into your life and say good-bye to it forever. It is so crucial that you make the life choices necessary to maximize your energy and wellness on an on-going and daily basis. Use the tools I am offering you. **Nurse, heal thyself.**

Notes

[1]Hans Selye quote retrieved June 20, 2005 from the American Institute of Stress Web site, http://www.stress.org

[2]Hans Selye's paperwork analogy comes from Bobbi R. Stevens, PhD. (2001), *Unlimited Futures: How to Understand the Life You Have and Create the Life You Want,* Naples, FL: Tara Publishing.

[3]Arlene Watrobski, BSN, RN, CEN, CCRN, in personal communication February 14, 2006.

References

American Psychological Association. (2005). Mind / Body Health: Did You Know. APA Help Center.

Retrieved June 20, 2005 from http://www.apa helpcenter.org/articles/article.php?id=103

Rosch, Paul J., MD. (n.d.). Reminiscences of Hans Selye, and the birth of "Stress." American Institute
of Stress. Retrieved October 20, 2005 from
http://www.stress.org/mementos.htm

Rosenstein, Alan H., MD, MBA. (2002). Nurse-
physician relationships: Impact on nurse satisfaction and retention. *American Journal of Nursing 102*(6), 26-34.

Selye, Hans. MD, PhD. (1950). *The Physiology and Pathology of Exposure to Stress; a treatise based
on the concepts of the general-adaptation-
syndrome and the diseases of adaptation.* Mont-
real: Acta.

Selye, Hans, MD, PhD. (1978). *The Stress of Life: The
famous classic – completely revised, expanded,
and updated with new research findings* (2nd
ed.). New York: McGraw-Hill.

6

Ineffective Coping

"All the things I really like to do are either illegal,
immoral, or fattening." – Alexander Woollcott[1]

I know a lot about this one. I suspect that, if you
are reading this book, you do too. As nurses, we are
constantly caring for others. We can't *not* do it. **The
problem arises when we are not taking care of ourselves**. The very thing that makes us good nurses –
our compassion and drive to help others – is the very
thing that often puts us last on our list of priorities. We
find ourselves disheartened and losing our way in a
struggling profession that we once loved, *and* forgetting
to make time for ourselves. We need to turn our healing
inward. We need to *HealThy Nurse.*

Nurses are notorious for what I like to call the
"*Over-* Syndrome." Many of us are *over*-worked, *over*-
weight, *over*-stressed, *over*-tired, and *over*-using alcohol, cigarettes, food, or any number of things. I realize
that there are some of you out there who react to stress
by not eating and over-exercising, but I am secretly

jealous of you, and I wouldn't know a thing about that. Rest assured though, that the principles are all the same. As nurses, we know, probably better than anyone, how bad all of these things are for our health and well-being. How many of us have helped a C.O.P.D. patient, whose body is ravaged after years of smoking, and who is struggling to breathe, all the while thinking, *"I need a cigarette!"*? We laugh about it among ourselves – part of that cynicism that allows us to survive. But what we really need is relief from the stress and time and space for ourselves.

While it is true that the profession itself doesn't cause us to over-eat, under-exercise, or do any of the things we know are bad for us, stress does lead us to make bad decisions. Remember, when we are over-stressed, our judgment and decision-making ability are impaired. Long hours plus staff shortages plus few, if any, breaks often equals fast food and sluggish mind / body systems. We *know* we need to exercise and eat right in order to fuel our bodies for maximum energy and to keep our tickers strong. We know the *what* and the *why* and even the *how*. It is the actual *doing* where we often fall short.

Let's face it, chocolate and a Diet Coke® are a hell of a lot more comforting than an apple, a handful of nuts and water. We convince ourselves that we do not have time to pack a healthy meal, exercise, get enough sleep, or treat ourselves to a massage. We tell ourselves that we have "earned" that cigarette, or that day-old piece of pie from the cafeteria that really didn't taste as good as you thought it would, but you could hardly tell because you only had three minutes to eat, pee, and call home to make sure everyone was still alive.

The reality is that so much of what we do to cope and to escape and to relieve stress is actually causing more pain. What we do may be instantly gratifying and may make us feel "better" for a moment, but these emotionally reactive coping mechanisms ultimately lead to feeling more tired, more sluggish, more pained, and maybe even a little guilty – with a dose of self-loathing thrown in for good measure.

Escapism in our society is at an all time high. But many of the

> *Until we get brutally honest about what we are really doing to cope, why it is counterproductive, and what we can do in place of those ineffective behaviors, we can't begin to make things better – for ourselves or for our patients.*

socially acceptable things we do to relieve stress or relax actually do just the opposite. Too often, we do not even realize that what we are doing to cope or get by is actually self-destructive and causing more stress and more pain. And if we do realize it, we are often too busy or too tired to make a change. We put it off for another day, another year, another lifetime. However, until we get brutally honest about what we are really doing to cope, why it is counterproductive, and what we can do in place of those ineffective behaviors, we can't begin to make things better – for ourselves or our patients.

We learn so much in nursing school. We study anatomy, physiology, and chemistry. We learn how to start an IV and how to make a bed with a nice neat corner (do they actually still teach that these days?). What we *don't* learn, and what we should make damn sure our new nurses *do* learn, is how to cope with what really lies ahead. Nursing can be an immensely rewarding and meaningful career. However, unless we provide ourselves, each other, and future nurses with the real-life powerful strategies necessary to *effectively* cope with the requisite stresses of the job, all the skills in the world won't mean a thing.

Notes

[1]Alexander Woollcott quote from R. E. Drennan (1973), *Wit's End*, retrieved October 6, 2005 from http://www.quotationspage.com/quote/30296.html

7

What I Learned & How it can Change Your Life

"Go confidently in the direction of your dreams!
Live the life you've imagined."
– Henry David Thoreau[1]

I remember thinking that if I felt all right and I wasn't sick, that I was healthy. I could not have been more wrong. The truth is that good health is more than just the absence of illness. Although I had discovered so much in the months leading up to this book and was excited to share what I had learned with other nurses, I realized that I was still angry. I was angry because I felt as though I had been forced to leave a position that I was good at and that I once loved.

I had been blaming my burnout on a nursing shortage out of control, politics, and bad management. But the truth was that **I had to take responsibility** for what had happened to me over the years, and I had to realize that I was *reacting* rather than *choosing* in all areas of my life. I kept hearing my mother's voice in the back of my head saying, *"It does no good to whine about something if you don't get off your ass and do something about it!"* I knew she was right.

Since Western medicine primarily focuses on what is wrong with people, I have always been intrigued by Dr. Abraham Maslow and his study of wellness and self-actualization. He found that self-actualized people are physically, emotionally, and spiritually healthy. They are greatly intuitive, creative, objective, and autonomous. The self-actualized person is spontaneous and prefers simplicity and nature. She is able to embrace solitude, is accepting of herself and others, and enjoys a very robust state of emotional and physical well-being. Dr. Maslow understood and acknowledged the importance and *inseparability* of the mind-body relationship.

Countless books have been written on the subject of self-actualization, and the term has even become a bit of a cliché. But I had always yearned for that enlightenment. I wanted to be that person sitting on top of the mountain, meditating for hours – never mind that I would be hard pressed to quiet my mind for two seconds. I longed to be at one with the universe and confident that all was right with the world. Ah! Imagine the serenity! And that was about all I did – imagine it. It is easy to become overwhelmed with all that self-actualization implies. I would make little attempts along the way – dutifully writing down my affirmations, and vowing to exercise and eat right and meditate and write a novel, and go ahead and create world peace while I was at it.

In the months leading up to my last day in the Emergency Department, my brother gave me a book by Bobbie Stevens, PhD, entitled *Unlimited Futures: How to Understand the Life You Have and Create the Life You Want.* That turned out to be another pivotal moment in my journey. Bobbie Stevens' notion of high-level wellness and the possibility of a "Superlife" struck me. I wasn't certain what it meant, exactly, but it sure sounded good. I began to study my life and really look at what I was creating. I learned that, like it or not, I was responsible for creating my own life. Moreover, my downward spiral towards depression and burnout was not just simply the result of politics or bad management or a nursing shortage out of control as I once thought. I was reminded that every choice has a consequence. **And when we decide not to choose, we have still made a choice.** We are giving someone else the power to make our decisions for us, and we still have to suffer the consequences. Ouch.

I began to realize, after a lot of soul searching, a lot of tears, and a few "a-ha!" moments, that I could create whatever I wanted in my life. We all can. And, while it may seem daunting (not to mention a little bit hokey) at first, it is really so simple. I finally began to embrace what Granny had figured out a long time ago, and what human potential sages have been teaching for centuries.

Meditate for 30 minutes twice a day? Not to mention the yoga, stretching, and affirmations? Yeah, right. Like I had time for that! I had a job (at least for a little longer), a toddler, a husband working full time and in graduate school, and a house to keep. Never mind all the hobbies and outside interests I vaguely recalled once having.

But once I let go of my "all or nothing" mentality of self-actualization and realized that self-actualization is simply a *choice* about how I live my life, I was free. I became determined to consciously choose, *to commit* to living my life with my whole soul – purely and joyfully. I learned that there *is* a perfect connection between the mind, body, emotions, and spirit.

Once I embraced the fact that self-actualization is an on-going process and that the beauty is that we never reach the top of that mountain, things began to shift. We are in such a hurry to create the perfect life *now*, that we often miss the fun and the journey of it. It starts out so small, with little steps. For instance, I began to look at meditation differently. Ideally, I would create time and complete silence for myself throughout the day to meditate, stretch, visualize – all the things that have been proven over centuries to work. But I don't always have time to myself in the morning. I can, however, help my daughter throw on her darling little leotard, and pop in a Pilates DVD. Before I know it, I'm focusing on my breathing, my body, my energy, and I can feel the stress melting away. We are quietly in sync, and I am connecting with my true self as well as my beautiful daughter. That's meditation to me.

When I finally let go of my "all or nothing" mentality of self-actualization and I realized that self-actualization is simply a choice about how I live my life, I was free.

I became determined to consciously choose, to commit to living my life with my whole soul – purely and joyfully.

I learned that there truly is a perfect connection between the mind, body, emotions, and spirit.

As I practiced what I was learning and embarked on this project, I could feel my life shifting. I was already taking much better care of myself. I naturally ate better and began walking (again, take your meditation where you can get it), and took to heart some basic principles. I had already made the choice to live whole-souled. I understood the power of choice and that we can either accept or reject negative energy. That, combined with truly embracing the understanding that you can't change others, made a tremendous difference.

I practiced "physualization," therapeutic breathing, and something I refer to as "let it go" to release tension and stress. I took "time outs" and breaks as I needed them, both at work and at home. The results were dramatic and amazing. I went from being completely miserable in my job to thinking that I could reframe it all, and enjoy it again. By this time, I was convinced that what I had learned could help any nurse

> *It is exciting – tremendously exciting – to discover that changing your entire life begins with no more than a small shift in your thinking!*

who was struggling with burnout and yearning for that ever elusive healthy life / work balance. I became determined to share what I had learned with others.

It is tremendously exciting to discover that changing your entire life begins with no more than a small shift in your thinking. The principles and strategies in *HealThy Nurse* are not earth-shattering or even new, but they *do* work. We live in an era when we are bombarded by the latest craze and one quick fix after another. I find it refreshing that what we are really searching for is already out there and that it was discovered centuries ago. If you have the time to read hundreds of books and years to figure out what works for you, then this book may not be for you. However, if time is at a premium in your life right now, this is exactly the right book for you. In the Emergency Department, you have to know a little about a lot of things. In other words, you don't have to know everything, if you know the right thing. Likewise, if you know the guiding principles of healthy successful living, you do not need to know the rest. Welcome to the right thing.

Notes

[1]Henry David Thoreau quote retrieved July 25, 2005 from http://www.quotationspage.com/quotes/Henry_David_Thoreau/

References

Stevens, Bobbie R., PhD. (2001). *Unlimited Futures: How to Understand the Life You Have and Create the Life You Want.* Naples, FL: Tara Publishing.

Component II.
The HealThy Nurse
Transformation Process™

The Core Concepts

Concept 1

Answer Your Own Call Light First

"Solitude is not a luxury. It is a right and a necessity."
– Anne Wilson-Schaef,[1] *Meditations for
Women Who Do Too Much Journal*

We have all heard that we need to fill our own cup first. It brings to mind the flight attendant who reminds us that, should we lose cabin pressure (that can't possibly be good) and those little masks fall from the ceiling, we should give ourselves oxygen before attending to the children and elderly on board. It seems crazy to think that I would let my daughter sit there without oxygen as I fiddle with my own mask. But when I really think about it, I am no good to her if I'm dead. The same goes for us as nurses. We must nurture our own minds, bodies, and souls *first.* We will, in turn, be happier, healthier, and better prepared to deal with whatever life throws at us. We will be better nurses, mothers, daughters, coaches, friends, and whatever else we want to be.

As we make our way through this life, we are taught to believe that if we are good, giving, and caring we will in return be happy, loved, and fulfilled. Unfortunately, we are inevitably left feeling disappointed or unworthy when our reality does not meet our expectations. When asked, most will say that they became nurses "to help people." The hard truth is that we cannot *help* anyone. We cannot heal them. We can only *assist* them in their healing. The only person that you can truly heal is *yourself.*

Whether we admit it or not, most nurses believe that taking care of others is somehow more honorable or noble than taking care of themselves. We often strive to keep the peace, and we avoid conflict at all costs. Many of us have difficulty setting boundaries. We have a hard time saying no. Nurses often find themselves in codependent or abusive relationships. We all know nurses (perhaps you are one of them) who are constantly putting out fires and managing crises, both at work and at home, while allowing their own health and happiness to suffer. Unfortunately, all of this leads to more stress, which can lead to feelings of helplessness, resentment, self-loathing, and any number of unhealthy or addictive behaviors – all in a misguided attempt to relieve our stress, alter our mood, or medicate our pain.

As the previous chapter revealed, stress can have a devastating effect on our mind / body / soul system. **When our minds and bodies are overwhelmed with stress, we are not able to see solutions to our problems.** As a result, we make poor decisions. Obviously, this creates bigger problems. The cycle continues, often without our even being aware, until we lose our true selves – along with our hopes, dreams and happiness.

What I am asking you to do will probably make you uncomfortable at first. **I challenge you to *put yourself first.*** Make your own needs a priority. Make time for yourself. Maybe that means learning to say "no" (without feeling guilty!). Maybe that means simplifying your life. Maybe that means just giving yourself permission. My point is this: **you must feed your soul**. What excites you? What are you passionate about? Rediscover those things. Or try something new.

If you won't give yourself permission, then take it from me. Why should you listen to me? Because I have been there. I know firsthand how putting yourself last, and not listening to that inner voice, damages your body and your spirit. I know what it feels like to lose yourself in everyone else's drama. I also know what it feels like to rediscover yourself and take your life back. Everyone should have that opportunity. Everyone should be able to live with her *whole* soul. Life is so grand, and we only get one shot. Take it!

Remember that it takes courage to do something radically different and to make the commitment to stem the assault and to start putting yourself first. You *can* be nurturing and giving. You *can* be an amazing nurse. But you can be these things without being a doormat or losing yourself along the way. Answer your own call light first. You simply have to commit to doing some very basic things for yourself on a daily basis. Remember that your focus is on progress, not perfection. By gradually expanding your awareness, you will open the door to true change.

Notes

[1]Anne Wilson-Schaef quote from Anne Wilson-Schaef (1992), *Meditations for Women Who Do Too Much Journal (*no pagination), New York: Harper Collins Publishers.

Concept 2

The Boomerang Principle

"Mind moves matter." – Virgil[1] (70-19 BC)

My daughter loves playing with the boomerang from her daddy's native Australia. As I watched her playing with it one day, I was struck by a thought. In this universe, this world, this life, it really is true that *what goes around comes around.*" Like so many of the age-old principles and concepts that ring true today, we are all familiar with this one. We just don't always apply it. The Boomerang Principle is my version of the Golden Rule, "What goes around comes around," or "Seek and you shall find."

Before we go any further, we must first review some very basic but universal laws and truths. Admittedly, this is the part where most self-help and personal growth books lose me, and I head for the fridge. But stay with me on this one. Very simply, we are all energy. Whether you consider it metaphorically or scientifically, this is one universal truth that has existed throughout time and in every culture. Call it what you will – energy, karma, mojo, etc. This has nothing to do with religion or myth or dogma. Basically, we are all connected to each other because we all come from the same source of light, love, and energy. Through our thoughts and actions, we are constantly giving out energy and attracting energy – whether we are conscious of it or not.

The bottom line is that **whatever we focus on is what we will create for ourselves.** The good news is that we get to choose what we give and what we receive. Nothing can be given if it's not accepted. You must decide what you will receive. This includes negative energy – whether from your past programming (our beliefs that result from past experiences), an annoying co-worker, or the ten-car pile up that is keeping you from getting wherever you need to be on time. But you can choose *not* to accept negative energy and focus only on accepting positive energy.

For instance, if we are constantly focusing on the problems in our lives, we will surely attract more problems. How many times have you been having a bad day with one thing going wrong after another? After a while, we begin to expect bad things to happen, and we're not surprised when they do. If we believe that we are unhappy, stressed out, or that we will have a bad day, then that will be our experience. If we focus instead on the positive and what we want to create in our lives, then *that* will be our experience. Remember that we receive what we put forth.

Remember, too, that negative energy is infectious. We can pass it on to others, just as they can pass it on to us – if we let them. Negative energy is *wasted energy.* It does absolutely no good to wish things were different, to lament about the past, or to whine and complain. It is all about choice. You must *choose* to change your life today. **The only time in existence is here and now.** It is both comforting and thrilling to know that, when we grasp and practice these simple concepts, it puts us in direct control of our experiences, thoughts, energy, and ultimately, our *lives.*

On the flip side, it is not enough just to choose not to receive negative energy. We must also be capable of receiving what it is we desire in our lives. This can be a tricky one since many of us struggle with self-worth issues and wonder if we are good enough or deserving enough. But trust that you are! With the concepts and strategies introduced in the coming chapters, through expanding your awareness and embracing your power to chose, you will naturally let go of all the self-defeating thoughts and habits that hold you back. You will learn to gradually replace them with healthy, positive, life-affirming thoughts and habits.

One of the most important aspects of the boomerang principle is gratitude. Whatever or whoever your source of light, love, energy, or intelligence is, remember to always give thanks. It is critical to stay connected with your source of abundance. The Boomerang Theory will help you do just that. By living and leading by example, you are automatically showing gratitude. Giving thanks is such an important piece – an often-overlooked piece – of that perfect connection between mind, body, emotions, and spirit.

Do you want less stress, more time, and a fulfilling and balanced life? Done! **Simply commit to *choosing* a different path**. Be just a little more courageous than you were yesterday. Choose to give positive energy. Choose to accept positive energy. Begin by making a few shifts in your thinking and a few changes in your life. Before long, almost effortlessly, you will start to live happier, healthier, better – with your whole soul. You choose. What kind of energy will *you* share with the universe?

[1]Virgil quote retrieved July 25, 2005 from http://www. brainyquote.com/quotes/quotes/v/virgil145496.html

Concept 3

Expand Your Awareness
(Optimal Awareness)

"Inspiration comes very slowly and quietly."
– Brenda Ueland,[1] *Mediations for Women
Who Do Too Much Journal*

As we observed in our discussion about the Boomerang Principle, we direct energy through our thoughts and thus, directly affect our reality. Whatever we focus on and believe about ourselves and our world is what we will create, be it positive or negative. A belief is really **nothing more than a picture in our mind that we have accepted as fact**. During our discussion about the Nurse's Dilemma, we noted how our beliefs or pictures tend to create many of our experiences, which in turn, validate our beliefs. (Dizzy yet?) This is why we tend to create many of the same life experiences for ourselves over and over. Weight loss attempts fail again? Always manage to get involved with the wrong guy? Kids seem to never listen? If we believe that our job is too stressful to handle or that we are incompetent, then *that* will be our experience. If you believe, "I am a shit magnet," then you will be. It's your self-fulfilling prophecy being fulfilled over and over again.

So, if our thoughts create our reality, then it follows that it is not a *situation* in itself that causes our suffering. It is our *thinking* about the situation that causes it. The next step is to begin the process of discovering what is really inside of us creating our thoughts and thus, our reality.

The truth is that so many of us are emotionally reacting to our lives and living unconsciously. Without even realizing it, we let situations from the past completely dictate our reactions in the present. The problem arises when so much of what we believe to be true and a matter of fact actually stems from negative experiences that originate as far back as childhood. These pictures or programming from our past and the rigid beliefs that have resulted are very often disempowering and limiting.

Life would be so much easier if we entered adulthood with nothing but programs or pictures of love, acceptance, empowerment, and total acceptance. I had (and thankfully still have) wonderful, loving, and supportive parents. I have lived a very fortunate and blessed life by all accounts, yet I have struggled to overcome my own self-limiting beliefs. We all must.

As a parent, I find this to be perhaps the most daunting challenge. How do I keep the rest of the world from getting to my little girl? Obviously, I cannot. I can, however, give her the best foundation I possibly can and do my best to make sure that she knows that she is positively and unconditionally loved, and that she is beautiful, strong, and brilliant just the way she is.

I can teach her to believe in herself and her power to *choose* and to *create* whatever she wants in her life. I can lead by example, and I can let her know that her thoughts and beliefs and therefore, her *life* are absolutely in her control. I can guide her. But ultimately, it is her journey, and she will have to learn and grow and figure it out on her own.

It takes a tremendous amount of courage to face and transcend our past programming and the resulting self-limiting beliefs. But if I can do it, you can too. Anyone can.

For those of you who have suffered serious emotional or physical abuse or rape, or have experienced other deeply traumatic events, the principles and strategies in *HealThy Nurse* absolutely apply, but you may need help beyond just a good book.

The bottom line is that **true change cannot come without awareness.** Getting brutally honest about what we are really doing to cope with stress and burnout, and why it is ineffective and even dangerous, can be both scary and painful. But it is also the crucial first step in expanding your awareness and starting that journey towards a healthier, happier, whole-souled life.

If you can change your limiting, non-supportive thoughts, habits, and actions, I promise you the payback will be immense. You have the power to respond from your higher self, rather than reacting from your programmed or fear-based self. If you want your world to be a certain way, then you must start with *you* being that way.

Once you start to become more aware of your negative thoughts, feelings, and actions, and you recognize them

> *It can be scary to admit that what you are doing to cope with stress and burnout is ineffective and even dangerous.*
>
> *But doing so is the crucial first step to expand your awareness and start that journey towards a healthier, happier, whole-souled life.*
>
> ***If you can change your limiting, non-supportive thoughts, habits, and actions, I promise you the payback will be immense.***

for what they are – simply beliefs or pictures that you have blindly accepted as fact over the years, you can then begin to move towards the next step, which is reconditioning or retraining your mind to respond supportively and positively to whatever challenges you face. The goal is to expand your awareness gradually, so that you can begin to live your life *consciously*. **The reality is that believing something doesn't necessarily make it true.** Those negative absolutes aren't so absolute anymore. Once you begin to expand your awareness and see your beliefs and pictures for what they really are, reframing and retraining your thoughts will be a very natural, almost effortless process.

To begin, I recommend starting a journal as you head into the following chapters. Journaling can be one of the most therapeutic forms of releasing stress, visualization (physualization), and taking "time out." It also promotes self-awareness. A simple notebook will do, but use something special if you prefer. This is *your* ritual. Do it in a quiet comfortable place. I have found that sitting and writing in nature as much as possible expands my awareness further and greatly improves the meditative qualities of journaling.

You will find that writing in your journal and revisiting what you have written will become enjoyable, relaxing, and something you will look forward to. Write down anything and everything in your journal.

Remember that it is private, and no one else has to see it. In fact, you can keep it under lock and key if it makes you feel better.

Journaling to expand your awareness

- *First*, **start to think about your own self-limiting thoughts and beliefs.** Write them down. Think about things you aren't happy with or want to change in your life. Look for self-defeating thoughts or programs, especially those that begin with *"I always..."* or *"I can't...,"* and *"A equals B"* worst-case-scenarios. As you become more aware, you will notice more and more of these self-defeating thoughts. You will also notice them in others. By simply becoming aware, you are making great strides.

- *Second*, **consider what you are really doing to cope with stress and burnout in your life.** Think about both your physical and emotional actions. For instance, I convinced myself for years that I was a "social smoker." (Does smoking in the company of your dog count?) Again, make a list. Seeing what you really do not want to face on paper somehow makes it more real.

- *Third*, **start to think about what you really want to create in your life.** Forgetting the how and when, and regardless of how unrealistic or far-fetched it may seem, write down your wildest dreams. What is your true purpose or calling in life? Are you living it? Make a list. Remember, whatever we believe and focus on is what we will create in our lives. You choose.

Once you begin to utilize a few of the basic concepts and strategies provided in the following chapters, you will automatically find more resourceful and supportive ways of living and being in your world – including the stressful and challenging nursing world. With commitment and practice, your expanded awareness will transfer into every other aspect of your life. Your world will naturally begin to shift towards a healthier, happier one. You will start to live consciously rather than unconsciously, and begin that fabulous journey up the mountain. Enjoy!

Notes

[1]Brenda Ueland quote from Anne Wilson-Schaef (1992), *Mediations for Women Who Do Too Much Journal,* (no pagination), New York: Harper Collins Publishers.

Concept 4

The Power of Choice

"Nothing is more difficult, and therefore, more precious, than to be able to decide."
– Napoleon Bonaparte[1]

As I mentioned earlier, every choice has a consequence. Like it or not, even if you decide not to choose, you still must experience or, worse, *suffer* the consequences. Many people never have the opportunity to truly choose what they want to be or to create in their life. Because we are so mired in our past programming, we live much of our life unconsciously, just going through the motions. We do what we have always done, regardless of how well it's working for us. This unconscious or reactive living leads to stress and burnout, and it prevents us from living with our whole soul.

Alternatively, we can *choose* to create a lifestyle that relieves stress on a daily basis, so that we are free to live with more health, happiness, and fulfillment. **When we are not over-burdened with stress, we are**

able to see clearly and solve our problems –
whether it is an immediate conflict on the job or a bigger, more daunting problem at home. The rest will take care of itself. When we *choose* to live consciously and unburdened by stress, we are open to everything that life and the universe have to offer. The truth is that anything we desire is attainable. We just have to *choose* what we really want in our lives. Once we begin this process of living consciously, we will naturally begin to see more clearly. We will effortlessly be drawn to the things that are good for our minds and bodies, and to the people who make us happy and complete. We will begin to live with our whole soul.

Changing your life, and opting for health and happiness instead of stress and despair, begins with a simple shift in thinking. That may sound overly simplistic, but it really is that easy. Simply making the choice – *the commitment* to embrace a few universal truths and to live a lifestyle that relieves stress on a daily basis – can and will drastically change your life, both at work and at home.

Recognizing that you have the power to choose whether you accept or reject positive and negative energy is instantly liberating. Of course, this does not mean that you live blindly or that you pretend the difficult things in life do not exist. But rather, you can choose how you react to what life throws at you, and you can choose to see things for what they really are, rather than the over-blown dramas your stressed-out mind tends to conjure up.

From cranky patients to the co-worker who always seems to drag down morale to the guy who cuts you off in traffic – you choose. By practicing a few simple strategies, you can choose to reject – or not internalize and embrace – the "small stuff." You can become better equipped to deal with those truly hard times if you are not already so emotionally exhausted and burned-out after holding on to the day to day stresses that build up and create barriers to true health and happiness.

I am notorious for beating myself up over past mistakes and worrying about the future. I knew I was a good nurse, but after making one med error, I was never the same. The error was benign – if there is such a thing as a benign med error. No one was even close to being hurt, and I learned to be even more vigilant as a result. Still, I could not forgive myself, and I could not get past it. But when I finally embraced the fact that **the**

past and the future do not exist except in my thoughts, I was able to move on. This does not, of course, mean that I am not responsible or accountable for my actions. But it allows me to let go of the thoughts, pains, fears, or worries that hold me back. **It is here and now where our power resides,** and that is a wonderful thing.

There is another component to the power of choice that we must be aware of – the often-frustrating reality that **you cannot make choices for others**. This can be a particularly hard truth for nurses to accept. For instance, we advise our cardiac patients that they need to stop smoking, eat properly, exercise, and take their meds. Yet, we are shocked and almost take it personally when they do not heed our advice and thus, return over and over again with the same complaints. Ultimately, we have to recognize and embrace the fact that we can offer our patients sound medical advice and excellent care, and we can provide them with the tools to live longer healthier lives. But we cannot force them to be more responsible, more accountable, or more compliant. **Just as we have the power to choose, so do they.**

The same holds true for our co-workers, managers, disgruntled patients, and the rest of the world for that matter. For instance, when we have a conflict with a co-worker, we can choose only how *we* will react. The tendency is to choose a struggle (whether we realize we have chosen it or not) and try to convince the other person that he or she is wrong and we are right. But with this choice, a struggle is pretty much all that we will experience. And more tension and more stress are sure to be the end result. Remember, they get to choose as well.

If we fall into the trap of expecting others to see things the way we do, whether it is our patients, our co-workers, or the rest of the world, we will invariably be disappointed. Once we embrace the power of choice – *for everyone* – we no longer have the need to convince anyone that we are right. Like the other principles, once we embrace **the power of choice**, it puts us in direct control of our world and what we create for ourselves.

Notes

[1]Napoleon Bonaparte quote retrieved July 25, 2005 from http://www.brainyquote.com/quotes/quotes/n/napoleonbo161724.html

Concept 5

You Can't Change Others

"Who looks outside, dreams; who looks inside, awakes." – Carl G. Jung[1] (Swiss psychologist)

When we surrender to the fact that we cannot change others, we realize that **we will be disappointed when we expect other people to see things as we do.** As we discussed in the previous chapter about the Power of Choice, it can be challenging and frustrating to admit that we cannot make choices for others. But it can also be a relief. When we commit to living with our whole soul – fully and honestly – we have no need to convince anyone else that we are right or that our way is the best way. When we embrace our power to choose, and we understand that everyone else has the same power, we realize that what is right for us may be wrong for another. It is all about acceptance. As nurses, we may know what *is* right, or at least *better,* for our patients, but ultimately, we cannot force them to recognize it, and they must make the choice themselves. We can, however, offer guidance, support, care, and an open heart – without being too attached to the end result.

One of the most painful and frustrating examples of this concept is the battered woman. Sadly, I have taken care of countless battered women over the years, and my heart has ached for each one of them. I can still see many of their faces, but one stands out in particular. She was a bright, beautiful young woman who came in repeatedly after her boyfriend would get drunk and beat her until she was nearly unrecognizable. I would help stitch her wounds, set her bones, and clean her up. I'd spend hours with her while my co-workers covered my other patients. I would fill out the requisite paperwork, organize a shelter, and send her friend to pack a bag. Each time, I was sure I had gotten through, thinking *"this time it's going to be different."* We would hug as she left my department and headed for the designated "safe place" and the help she needed.

Inevitably, she would return. I had studied battered women, and I understood the psychology of why they stayed. I could not get through to this woman. Even the threat of death was not enough. I was sad for her. And I was sad for her daughter. I knew the odds were against her little girl, and that, statistically, she would likely fall into the same trap and the cycle would continue. I felt helpless to stop it, frustrated, and angry. In spite of all the literature I had studied, and all the good I meant, I could not do a damn thing to keep this woman from going back to her abuser. And each time she returned to the ED – with injuries more severe than before – I would swear that this was the last time I'd let myself get emotionally involved. But alas, we are nurses, and we never stop trying.

That's where I got hung up on this one. It is all well and good to say that you can't change others, but so much of what we do as nurses is all about changing people. We help fix what's broken. It is what we do. Whether it's the alcoholic (who always claims he only had two beers and was just minding his own business), or the little old man who won't take his heart medication, or the diabetic whose diet is out of control, we cannot stop trying to get through to our patients. We can, however, cut ourselves some slack and *let go* of the end result. We must realize that we can provide them with the information and the tools. We can encourage and support them and even pray for them. But **we cannot change them.** They have to do that for themselves. They have to make the choice. Period.

This is not an *"I'm OK, you're OK"* book. And it is definitely *not* one of those self-help books that lets you and everyone else off the hook, reassuring you that nothing is really your fault. Indeed, it is just the opposite. **We are all *absolutely* accountable for the choices we make and lives we live.** We are all responsible for our own thoughts, actions, health, and happiness. We just have to recognize that we cannot force others (our patients) to be accountable or responsible. We cannot force them to see the error of their ways or to be even a little bit kind – try as we might. That's a big pill for nurses to swallow.

On another note, you may find that as you embrace more of these principles, and your life begins to shift, you will naturally be attracted to people who bring about more positive energy. Likewise, those who have more positive energy will likely be drawn to you.

Many people may find that relationships that once "worked" are no longer good for them. I am not out to shake up any marriages or to break up friendships. As we embark on this journey of self-discovery and happiness, we cannot help but get excited and want to share our excitement with those who mean the most to us. But the truth is that not everyone may be as enthusiastic as we are. They may feel threatened or simply are not ready to change their own lives. They may never be ready. When those people who are meant to be supportive and loving in your life attempt to sabotage your journey and happiness, you may naturally re-evaluate those relationships. Remember that, especially when faced with another person's doubt, it takes courage to be true to your self.

Notes

[1]Carl G. Jung quote retrieved July 25, 2005 from http://www.brainyquote.com/quotes/quotes/c/carlgjung1 32738.html

Concept 6

The Law of Replacement

"In as much as the soul is present, there will be power." – Ralph Waldo Emerson[1]

Like so many ideas I have introduced here, replacement is a simple enough concept. It is also where so many people fall short in really changing their lives. The idea of gradual replacement simply states that you must replace or exchange one behavior with another. Again, that's easier said than done. It is so easy to say, *"I'm going to lose weight"* or *"I'm not going to let work get to me today."* The truth is that **if we do not have a plan, we are going to fail.** I may be the world record holder for "fresh starts" and lofty resolutions. I have also failed at all of them because I didn't stand a chance. I beat myself up countless times until I finally realized the wisdom of replacement – **we must replace one bad behavior with another, healthy one.**

Think about it. Go back to the list you have been thinking about or writing in your journal. Review the behaviors, self-defeating thoughts, or things about yourself that you most want to change. Your list may include emotional eating, smoking, drinking, conflicts at work, or tension at home. Take a few minutes to study your list. Are you beginning to recognize that the behaviors, thoughts, and other things on your list are reactive, often unconscious, responses to stress?

We have all resolved at one time or another to stop doing something we know is either unhealthy or just plain making us miserable. The double whammy hits when you start out with the best of intentions, and maybe even all the will power in the world, only to find that you fail within the first day – sometimes the first hour – of your new lease on life. This, in turn, leads to a frustrating sense of failure, guilt, and a *"to hell with it!"* attitude of abandonment. My attempts at dieting are a classic example of this. I would start a new program, proclaiming *"Today is the first day of the rest of my life!"*, slip up (usually within several hours), and then throw caution to the wind and eat almost without pause for the rest of the day. This, of course, would lead me to feel even worse, and the vicious cycle would continue. It has been said that success depends on three things; genetics, luck and preparation. We have control over only one of those things. Or, as my father so eloquently reminds me, *"Good things happen by plan. Shit happens all by itself."* [2] The bottom line is that you have to take a few critical steps and **make a plan** in order to really change your behavior.

Make the Law of Replacement work for you

- *First,* **look at the behavior you want to change.** For instance, it is not enough to say, *"I'm going to eat healthy."* Be specific. What are you eating now? Does it fuel your body or make you sluggish and slow you down? Are you eating on the go? Are there not enough healthy options in the cafeteria? (It is shocking, by the way, how utterly unhealthy most hospital cafeteria fare is. *"Will it be starch, starch, or starch today, Nurse Carr?"*) Do you plan your meals or just grab what is handy?

- *Second,* **dig deep and consider *why* you engage in this harmful behavior.** Is it an emotional reaction to stress? Is it just something you have always done? Look at what gratification you get – at least immediately – from this behavior. Chances are good that it is some form of comfort or "pick-me-up." Think about the consequences. Realize how this behavior is actually making you feel worse in the long run.

- Take smoking, for instance. Most people who smoke will say they do it because it relaxes them. In truth, smoking does the exact opposite. It raises your heart rate and your blood pressure. It restricts airflow and taxes your body. It is the farthest thing from relaxing. Of course, as nurses we know all of this. It just goes to show how powerful these coping mechanisms can be and how hard they are to let go of. Over time, we become more and more stressed out about what we *know* it is doing to our health, the horrible death we are sure to face, *what will my kids do when I'm gone?* But if we really think about it, what we are really looking for is probably space and time to ourselves, a sense of control, and that (until now) ever-elusive relief from stress.

- *Finally,* **choose to** *replace* **your bad habit with another, healthy behavior.** Remember, expanding your awareness is key to discovering your self-defeating habits. You will then be able to more easily replace a life-destroying behavior with a life-affirming behavior. (I will talk more about healthy replacement behaviors in the following chapters.) Make a commitment to using one of the stress release methods that we will talk about rather than reacting unconsciously to that co-worker or the patient's family member who makes you want to scream or run to the fridge. Believe me, I never thought I would give up my after-work smoke for deep breathing and meditation, *but I have never felt better.* For inspiration, revisit the list of things you want to create in your life – your passions – or what you think you might like to get passionate about.

What most people who want to quit a bad habit or lose weight or change their life in any way often miss is that they must go inside, figure out *why* they are doing what they are doing, *commit* to changing their behavior, and *form a plan of action*. Will power alone just won't cut it. We have to "do the work" to expand our awareness and naturally dissolve the stress and disempowering beliefs and habits that keep us so stuck, anxious, and sick.

Once we make the conscious choice and commit to doing the work, we will gradually replace each bad habit or disempowering belief with a belief or habit that is positive and that serves us well. Remember that it is not an all or nothing challenge. Be kind to yourself. If you slip up, acknowledge it, pat yourself on the back for recognizing it, and move on. You will find that, as you implement more and more of these strategies and make them part of your daily routine, you will naturally and effortlessly let go of the un-resourceful and unhealthy behaviors that have been keeping you from relieving stress on a daily basis and ultimately, living with your whole soul.

Notes

[1]Ralph Waldo Emerson quote from Bobbie R. Stevens (2001), *Unlimited Futures – How to Understand the Life You Have and Create the Life You Want* (p. 87), Naples, FL: Tara Publishing.

[2]My father, David Gregory.

Concept 7

It Takes Courage to Live With Your Whole Soul

"May you live every day of your life."
– Jonathan Swift[1] (1667-1745)

All the concepts we have discussed are simple and come from a great many years of study, self-discovery, and committed practice. They are universal laws. They are not rocket science. Yet, if you can fully embrace these few simple concepts, you can radically change the way you view the world and your place in it. This includes your role as a nurse.

Unfortunately, many of these universal laws, while common sense, are not widely accepted and certainly are not commonly practiced. Our society tells us that we must go-go-go and that the bottom line is the top dollar. We are constantly bombarded by the media and by our own self-defeating thoughts telling us that we have to move faster, do more, and be more – super bod, super parent, super career woman, super *every*-thing.

The same holds true in nursing. We are generally working with a shoestring staff and on an even smaller budget. Many of us work long hours, do not get breaks, and, if we do, often feel that we cannot take them. We are individually and collectively tired, lost, and burned-out. We do not have the tools to effectively cope with the everyday stresses of life and the strain of a nursing industry spiraling out of control. We are so busy just trying to keep up, that we do not even realize how much the build-up of stress and fatigue damages our bodies, minds, and spirits. Remember that stress impairs our thought processes and prevents us from clearly seeing solutions to our problems. Small hiccups become big problems. We get angry or upset about things that would not bother us if our thoughts and hearts were clear and free.

You *can* change your life today. *This very instant.* You can make the choice to commit to a lifestyle that relieves stress on a daily basis and frees you to live your best life, with your whole soul. It takes courage to take the leap, but I promise you that it will be well worth the effort. The journey towards a healthy mind and body, and towards the ultimate life / work balance takes courage because you may be going against the grain. However, you must trust that you are on the right path – *your right path* – despite everyone else going down the same unconscious, unhealthy path towards self-destruction and unhappiness. Know that it is not always going to be an easy journey. It may, at times, be uncomfortable along the way and even a bit painful. That said, it might also be the most fun you have ever had.

Points to Remember Along the Way

First, start and end every day with something positive. How many of us wake up and immediately turn on the radio or the television? We do it without thinking because it is what we have always done. The first and last thing many of us hear each day is about all the death and despair in the world. Don't we get enough of that at work? Of course, our intention is usually to be connected with the rest of the world – to catch up. But why not *first* connect and catch up with yourself? Instead, start and end each day by treating yourself to some quiet, peaceful solitude. Review the focus items you developed through journaling, meditate, stretch, or practice any of the other *HealThy Nurse* strategies.

Second, remember that there is no final stopping point to your growth and evolution. Like it or not, we never do make it to the top of that mountain. And what a fabulous thing that is. If we raced to the top, we would miss out on the fun and beauty of the journey. So, lighten up and go easy on yourself. Never stop learning, growing, and evolving. Recognize your progress and that *you* created it.

Third, listen to your inner voice. Once you have the knowledge and the tools, you will not want to wait on others. You will naturally want to live with your whole soul; you will want to live and lead by example. You will automatically begin to create the ultimate life / work balance. It is your choice. Choose to be courageous!

Notes

[1]Jonathan Swift quote retrieved July 28, 2005 from http://www.brainyquote.com/quotes/quotes/j/jonathons w101069.html

The Core Strategies

Strategy 1

Physualize
(Beyond Visualization)

"Act as if...." – My Mother[1]

Visualization may be one of, if not *the most important* strategy for relieving stress, creating your own reality, and, ultimately, freeing you to make the journey up that mountain towards a truly happy life. It is the foundation for all the other strategies. Through *physualization,* we can learn to live with our whole soul.

As I've confessed, I have been known to hop on a few self-help bandwagons in my search for personal growth and happiness. These self-help plans all have had some component of visualization. But I have found that visualization is so much more than just affirmations and mantras. If you can look at yourself in the mirror and exclaim, *"I am happy!"* or *"I am relaxed!"* without laughing and get the results you want, then more power to you. But I always felt like I was trying to pull one over on myself with such proclamations. I couldn't ever drown out that little voice in the back of my head reminding me that I was not yet any of the things I had longed for. I also found that trying to visualize a babbling brook while getting yelled at by an irrational "customer" was of absolutely no use.

As with many of the other ideas we have touched on, there are volumes of information out there about visualization. Let me remind you again that you do not need to know everything *if you know what really works.* Once we begin to consciously expand our awareness, we become more aware of our self-defeating thoughts and beliefs. We can then begin to replace them with healthy positive thoughts and beliefs, and we can let go of the past. This puts us in direct control of our own experiences and our own future. We cannot create anything on the outside until we can create it on the inside. In other words, **if you are not truly living it on the inside first, you will never live it on the outside.**

Visualization has five key components:

1. **Courage and Clarity**
2. **Commitment**
3. **Internal Focus or *Physualization***
4. **External Declaration**
5. **Manifestation and Appreciation**

> 1. ***Courage and Clarity.*** First, *be courageous* when it comes to discovering what it is you really want to create in your life. Sit quietly and revisit the list you started earlier. Now get more specific. If you haven't already, make a list of your goals and dreams. Do not worry about how you will reach those goals, or how unrealistic they may seem. And do not focus only on monetary or materialistic things. Just think about what would make your soul happy. What kind of relationships do you want with yourself, your source, your partner, or your kids? *Get very clear* and go into as much detail as possible. What exactly would it look like, smell like, taste like, even *feel* like to have these dreams come

true? The more detailed you make your vision, the quicker it will manifest itself.

2. **Commitment.** The next step is *commitment*. It is not enough to simply want something. Everyone *wants*. Obviously, not everyone *gets*. Remember that the results we achieve in life are in exact proportion to the intensity and dedication of our commitments. **You must make a commitment to making what you desire come to be.** Committing yourself implies that you will go to whatever lengths necessary to see your vision become a reality and that you have ruled out all possibility of failure. *This minor shift in the visualization process is a very powerful and motivating force.* Once you are able to commit to what it is you really want – to see it and feel it already realized – you will automatically draw towards you the energy necessary to make it happen.

3. **Physualization or Internal Focusing.**
The third step is *Internal Focusing* or
Physualization. This is such a crucial
part of visualization, and it is where so
many books, programs, and gurus fall
short. Goddard Neville got it right when
he said, *"Assume the feeling of the wish
fulfilled."*[2] Visualization is more than just
wanting something or seeing it in your
mind. It involves *becoming* that vision.
You must *feel* it. Think about what you
want to be, do, or have, and then *feel* it.
Imagine it already accomplished and feel
the thrill of it as a reality. **Feel, smell,
taste, *be* that goal already reached.** After all, isn't it the *feeling* that we are all
really searching for? It's not really about
more money, the bigger house, the ideal
job, or any of the things we think we need
to make us happy or to relieve our stress
and anxiety. It is the *feeling* that we are
searching for. When we begin to cultivate
the feeling that we desire on the inside,
the internal energy that we will be creat-

ing will begin to attract the outside actions and situations that will make our wish or feeling a reality. Now *that's* empowering!

4. ***External Declaration.*** The fourth component is *External Declaration.* Mantras and affirmations are a helpful aspect of visualization, but be aware that simply having them or repeating them is not enough. You must *first* see and feel what you want on the inside. It is not enough to say, *"I want to lose weight"* or *"I want to be rich"* or *"I want to live stress-free."* Think about the specific things you might do to achieve your goals and dreams. *Physualize* them. Also, be sure to frame them well. For instance, do not say, *"I won't eat anything bad for me today."* Using the word "won't" focuses on the negative. Instead, put a positive spin on whatever it is you are committed to doing or being. You might try saying, *"I commit to eating only healthy food that feeds my body and fuels my mind."*

Physualize

As part of your visualization, it helps to write down your focus items, whatever they may be, and review them – *feel them* – regularly. I suggest twice a day, once in the morning and at some time in the evening before you go to bed. You need to figure out what works for you. It is easy to get lost and feel like a failure if you cannot keep up with the specific time frames and schedules that so many books or programs recommend, so I purposely do not make too many suggestions regarding when and how often you should practice the strategies. Part of choosing a lifestyle that releases stress on a daily basis includes *finding out what works best for you*. Having a rigid program or schedule only creates more stress in my book – no pun intended. Eventually, as your stress diminishes, your life will shift, and you will make more time to practice the strategies. You will look forward to it, and wonder how you ever lived without them.

5. **Manifestation and Appreciation**. The final component of visualization is *Manifestation* and *Appreciation*. Through physualization, you will gradually replace the old, negative pictures and feelings, which have created your world up until now, with new, positive pictures and feelings. Allow yourself to recognize and appreciate the fact that *you* have manifested these positive changes in your life. *You* have harnessed the energy necessary to create whatever it is you have committed to creating. Give thanks to yourself, the universe, and your source. Remember that boomerang.

As you think about what it is you truly want to create in your life, you will no doubt start to get excited about the future. You may also be a bit apprehensive or even fearful about getting your hopes up too high. I know I was. At first, the specifics might seem a little overwhelming, and you might wonder how in the world you are going to make your dreams a reality. Just remember that once you become more relaxed, and you begin practicing the other strategies, your mind will open up, and the answers will naturally flow. Once you are able to commit to what you really want to create in your life, and you feel it already realized, you will automatically draw the positive energy necessary to make it happen. Can it really be that simple? It is. But only if you believe that it is, and if you open your mind to all that the universe has to offer.

You may be thinking that this is all well and good in the big scheme of things, but *"how the *!#% is it going to help me when I'm in the trenches with more patients than I can manage and not enough help, and I'm running on four hours of sleep?!"* The answer is this: part of being able to deal with stress "in the moment" is having a healthy, relaxed mind and body to begin with. Remember the paperwork analogy. When we are over-stressed, our problems seem overwhelming. By practicing physualization, and by getting into a "good place" in the morning and evening, we are better prepared for the challenges of our day. We will be able to react *consciously* rather than reactively to stress.

Yes, stress will bombard us. We know that our industry is in trouble, and we are feeling the effects firsthand. We are *over-stressed* to say the least. And I am not talking about relieving the stress of a code here. Obviously, we need that stress response to save that life. In the coming chapters, I will address ways to relieve stress "in the moment." If visualizing that babbling brook helps, then use it. Or, when you feel (note I said *feel*) stress taking over, try one of these other physualization strategies. Remember to combine the feeling with the picture or vision.

> Say: *"I **feel** myself relaxing right now, and I see myself handling this situation calmly and consciously."*

> Say: *"I **feel** myself breathing deeply right now."* At the same time, take a deep cleansing breath. As you exhale, *feel* the release of tension and stress.

Note that these are simple techniques – they may even seem silly at first glance. But however simple it may be, no strategy will work unless you actually commit to using it. The point is this: open your mind to new ways of living and relieving stress. With each accomplishment, you will become more confident, and more accomplishments will naturally follow. By practicing physualization on a regular basis, you will be better prepared to combat stress on a day-to-day basis and in the moment.

Notes

[1]My mother, Susie Gregory.

[2]Goddard Neville quote from Goddard Neville: Fundamentals, Cornerstone Books Web site, retrieved October 20, 2005 from http://nevillegoddard.www.hubs.com /neville1.htm

Strategy 2

Take Time Out

"Our life is frittered away by detail...
simplify, simplify."
– Henry David Thoreau,[1] *Walden*

Take time out for yourself. This is one of the crucial strategies that so many people – *especially nurses* – miss. We often, by nature, have difficulty saying no and setting boundaries. We are programmed to go-go-go, and we do not take scheduled breaks – *if* we get them at all. I was certainly guilty of this. There is no end to the workload, and it seems there is always more to do. Lunch breaks were simply not taken where I worked. We ate if and when we could, and it was always on the run. How many of us have caught ourselves while out for a lovely evening at a nice restaurant, scoffing our food down as our friends or family look at us as if we were animals? In addition, many of us work overtime because we feel obligated to our patients, our units, or for the all-mighty dollar. However, there are three things we all should do in order to drastically improve our lives and our practice: *take more breaks, simplify our lives, and get more sleep!*

Take More Breaks

I cannot stress enough the importance of getting *away*, getting *out,* and getting *air, sun, or sea.* The physiological and psychological benefits of taking time out are immense. I remember working 12-hour shifts (both days and nights) during the winter months. It was dark when I went to work and dark when I finished. Since I did not take any breaks, I would often go several days without seeing sunlight. I was, in a word, *miserable.* I couldn't quite put my finger on it, as I was working the same shifts and the same number of hours I always had. If only I had known then what I know now, that just taking time out and away from the unit to get outside, breathe some fresh air, and re-energize would have done wonders for me. Never dismiss the powerful effects of stepping away from that stressful environment, getting outside, and getting some air. Not only will you feel refreshed and revitalized, you will be better equipped to care for your patients. Learning to take time out is a crucial aspect to overhauling your work experience and your life.

On a broader level, taking scheduled breaks makes you much less likely to feel over-whelmed and over-stressed when things get hectic. If it is not common practice to take breaks where you work, talk to your manager. By law, employers are required to offer regular breaks to their employees. However, it is not enough to simply have a *policy* that allows breaks periodically. **If nurses do not feel that they can take breaks, it is the same as not allowing them at all.** Many of us do not take breaks because we feel that we don't have the time, or we fear that our workmates or managers will think less of us. If leadership in your department is resistant, take the lead yourself. I am not talking about a radical revolt or strike here. But we can all lead by example.

Not getting breaks is one of the chief complaints among today's nurses. As with so many other issues challenging nursing today, leadership is key. Managers, one of the best things you can do is to encourage your staff – *all* of your staff – to **take periodic breaks.** You

> *"Indeed, by improving the well-being of nurses, you can also improve the well-being of patients. Breaks increase nurses' productivity and efficiency and reduce accidents and errors."*
> – Flanagan (2005, p. 112)

will be rewarded with a much happier, more efficient staff that is less likely to burnout and more likely to stick around. Engage and *listen to* your staff to figure out what will work best for your unit. After all, they are the ones who really know the flow of that unit the best.

Nurses, you can work with each other to make sure that everyone gets periodic scheduled breaks. Get creative. Challenge yourselves to think outside the box and consider all the possibilities. Perhaps the manager could step in to cover patients from time to time throughout the day to allow for more breaks. Maybe it is worth considering a float or an extra staff nurse to cover patients periodically so that everyone gets an opportunity to take a break. Consider using charts or sign-up sheets. Draw from a hat. Do whatever it takes!

> **Nurse safety directly affects patient safety**
>
> *"Poor staffing can result in greater patient mortality. Mandatory overtime and long shifts can increase nurses' fatigue, stress, risk of accidents, and can impair work performance. When nurses and patients share the same environment, they share the same hazards, such as infectious agents, toxic cleaning chemicals, poor air quality, needlesticks, and violence."*
> – Flanagan (2005, p. 112)

Obviously, there are patient safety issues and standards of practice that must be considered. And we all know that budgets are tight. However, to survive and avoid burnout, we must gradually shift the thinking in our nursing culture. In order to provide the best care to our patients, we must answer our own call light first – which means taking time out during our shift to get away, get some air, and re-group. As far as those organizations who do not allow for a meal break within the normal paid work shift – especially a 12-hour shift – shame on you. Are we professionals or automated robots? Managers, by engaging, empowering, and encouraging your staff to take more breaks, you will be enhancing productivity and job satisfaction, and you will be boosting morale beyond what any survey, pep talk, or picnic could do.

Below I discuss three types of breaks that we should all incorporate into our workday. This means that you will know going into your shift that, no matter what it throws at you, you can make time – however brief – to get away from it all. Incorporating regular breaks will require cooperation from everyone concerned. Here are some suggestions to get the ball rolling.

- Do not wait for others to start the trend. Take the initiative.
- Remember the boomerang principle. Be certain that you return the favor when someone covers your patients while you take a break.
- Come up with a signal or clue among your co-workers that you can use to let each other know you are "off" and may need to de-stress and re-group.
- Offer to cover a colleague's patients for a few minutes, and encourage her to take a break if it appears as though stress is taking over. Sometimes when we are in the moment and overwhelmed, we cannot see how stress is affecting us. Reciprocity is essential for this change in thinking to manifest itself and for breaks to become more common in our work place.

Every nurse should have access to breaks during each and every shift she works. Our bodies need to re-fuel and rest. Our minds need to rest and de-stress. Even a few minutes can make all the difference. Work to incorporate all three of these types of breaks into your schedule:

1. **Scheduled Breaks (20 to 40 minutes).** Scheduled breaks should be a *minimum* of 20 minutes, and ideally, longer. This time is essential for *getting away from the unit*, sitting down, and eating a healthy meal or snack. This means that you do not need to scarf down whatever you can get your hands on right there in the nurse's station while standing up, giving report over the phone, and charting. Remember that you need to *re-fuel* your body, not drag it down. Get outside and breathe some fresh air, regardless of the temperature or time of day. Rug up if you have to. The jolt of crisp *fresh* air will do wonders for your psyche and your physical energy. Take a few minutes to practice any of the other strategies you find helpful – stretching, breathing, or meditating. Again, if this is unheard of on your unit, work to change the thinking.

2. ***Mini-Breaks (5 to 10 minutes).*** Aside from taking scheduled breaks, you can also take mini-breaks, time out to relieve stress in the moment. If you have a particularly stressful patient or a conflict with a co-worker, ask a friend or charge nurse to cover your patients for 5 to 10 minutes so that you can take a break. Remember to get away (within reason, of course) from the unit or the stressful situation and to get outside if you can. *Breathe.* Again, there are certain requirements for staffing and patient safety that need to be considered.

3. ***Time-Out (1 to 5 minutes).*** Time-out breaks can be used any time – particularly when you feel you do not have time to take a break. When stress is overwhelming you, and you cannot get away physically, re-member that you can still "get away." You can walk around the corner and just *breathe.* Get away from the situation with-out leaving your area. Do whatever you can to relax in that moment – breath, visu-alize, or stretch. It takes only a few sec-

onds to release stress and tension and be able to see things more clearly.

As we well know, it is not always "socially acceptable" in our field to take breaks. But if we can start to re-frame our work environment and encourage healthy coping mechanisms among our friends and colleagues, we will go a long way toward beating burnout. Remember that it takes courage to go against the grain. It might not be the most popular stance, but if we believe in what we are doing and lead by example, others will be at first curious, then intrigued, and then inspired to follow suit.

Another aspect of taking time out is the vacation. I know countless nurses (sadly, I was never one of them) who have accumulated hundreds upon hundreds of vacation or paid time off hours. Yet, they never use them. I often hear that they are saving those hours "for a rainy day." If you are reading this book, chances are good that that rainy day is here.

Remember that **one of the most important ways we can avoid burnout is to avoid exhaustion**. One way to do this is to take regular vacations. If your idea of a vacation is an exotic cruise or an African Safari that you cannot afford, then re-frame immediately! I am so fortunate in my life to have traveled to some very exciting and far away places. However, some of the most relaxing and refreshing vacations I have ever taken have been those in which I haven't traveled anywhere. The point is to get away from that stressful situation – your job or your normal routine – on a regular basis. If you cannot travel to another location, make your own retreat. Turn off the phone, the television, and the computer. Send the kids away – even if it is just for a few hours. Book a spa day or at least a massage. And here's a good one – *sleep.*

Make a "crash cart" for yourself. Fill a basket with your favorite scented candles, herbal teas, videos, bubble bath, music, or whatever makes you happy. Pull it out when you cannot get away, time is tight, or until you can take that cruise. Just knowing that crash cart is there waiting for you does wonders when your job feels like one big disaster after another. The point is not to wait to take a vacation. Do it now. Do it often. By avoiding exhaustion, you are avoiding burnout.

Simplify Your Life

As nurses, we are used to long shifts, over-time, and the cultural mind-set of go-go-go. Most of us are driven, at least to some degree, by money. Don't worry. I am not about to trail off into an *"all we really need is love"* spiel. I'm the first to say that I wish I had more money – *lots* more of it. Obviously, we need money to survive and to do some of the things that feed our soul. For instance, my husband and I love the ocean. We share the dream of living by the ocean one day. However, on a strictly practical note, property by the ocean is quite expensive. There is no amount of self-actualization or physualizing that will change that. Still, we are committed to seeing that dream realized, and I have no doubt that we will.

Working 12 to 16 hours is common in nursing and in many other facets of life these days. Over the years, I have worked every shift there is to work, and I feel that I can say with some authority that working 12-hour shifts is just not good for any of us. There have been countless studies showing that effectiveness and alertness decline in those last few hours, and that more mistakes are made in the last hours of a 12-hour shift. Additionally, it takes much longer to recover physically and emotionally after a 12-hour shift – especially as we get older. (I'm only 37, people. I shouldn't feel this old!!!) We *know* that working long hours can be dangerous to ourselves and to our patients. Nevertheless, we convince ourselves that we can handle it, that we won't make that med error, that we won't be the one to fall asleep behind the wheel, and that we would rather work more hours at a time and fewer days. Well, I propose that, by reassessing our lives and making a few minor and relatively painless adjustments, we can work fewer hours *and* fewer days.

Our society bombards us with images telling us that a better body, a bigger house, a better car, and sharper clothes all equal happiness. The truth is that if we are waiting for those material or physical things to make us happy, we are going to be waiting *forever*. I am guilty of thinking that if I could just reach my goal weight, everything would be right with the world, I would finally be happy, and my life would truly begin. I finally realized what a shame it would be to miss all that time in between – never mind that I was not able to reach that goal until I embraced the principles and strategies in *HealThy Nurse*. Just like that house on the ocean, if I wait until it becomes a reality to really start living my life, I will have missed so much of the ride.

I challenge you to really look at what you're spending your money on. How much do you spend on coffee or soda, cigarettes, fast food, or that pick-me-up snack from the vending machine every day? How often do you buy on impulse – another socially acceptable and encouraged way to escape the pain and stress in our lives? Don't get me started on the outrageous amount of consumer debt in this country ("*Refinance today! Simply sign here, and we'll own you for the rest of your life.*").

Do you really need cable or satellite TV? How does it affect you to start and end your day with violence and negativity – whether it is the morning news or yet another crime drama? More importantly, how does TV affect *your kids* (and what examples are you setting for them)?

Don't get me wrong. I love a good "Law & Order" or an old "Seinfeld" episode. And I don't believe there is any harm in losing ourselves briefly with a little healthy escapism. I am only suggesting that we become more aware of what we are *creating* in our lives. Perhaps we could watch less television and read more – engage our imaginations rather than bombard and overload our senses. After all, don't we get enough of that at work? What if we learned to sit in silence and to be comfortable with who we are in that silence?

This may sound like a contradiction, but if you look at your time in terms of money, you might be able to make more cutbacks. For instance, write down everything you spend in a week on the "extras" in your life, and tally it up. You may not look at that cup of Starbucks® on the way to work as an "extra" now – it may be all that's keeping you going. I am not even suggesting that you should give up coffee or Starbucks® all together. Just look consciously at what you are spending your money on. Remember, true change cannot come without awareness.

Now you can look at those non-essential items in terms of monthly or yearly expenditure. They add up! Consider how many hours you have to work to pay for those "extras." Are they really worth it? Maybe not so much. Perhaps you could be *not* working those hours, and instead, be doing something else that is your soul's preference. Just a thought.

Get More Sleep

Another important aspect of taking time out is *sleep*. Quite simply, we don't get enough of it. For whatever reason, 8 has become the accepted magic number through the years – although I have read that anywhere from 3 to 11 hours is acceptable. Personally, I tend to lean toward the 11 hours mark – which irked my father to no end as I was growing up *("Up at the crack of noon I see.")*. Who is the freak of nature that functions well on only three hours of sleep and makes the rest of us look like slackers?

We have all *existed* or *functioned* on three hours of sleep. But it is hard to imagine that anyone can feel well rested or perform at peak after only a few hours of sleep. The truth is that we all require different amounts of sleep throughout our lives, and there is no pre-scribed number of hours that suits us all. Sorry, Dad.

Each of us possesses an incredible, natural, internal stress-relieving system – *sleep.* Yet, most of us do not take advantage of this powerful gift. Instead, to the contrary, we all share some degree of sleep deprivation. Most of us would be overjoyed to get 8 hours of sleep these days.

Sadly, many of us get only a few solid hours of sleep each night. Our lives are so hectic that we just do not make time for sleep. Or, we are so wound up and our heads reeling from the stress of the day (or night) that sleep eludes us. Of course, yet another scenario is that you are nearly eight months pregnant as I currently am, and are up every two hours dashing to the bathroom.

Remember, one of the most important ways you can avoid burnout is to avoid exhaustion. Sleep, and getting enough of it, is essential for creating a life that relieves stress on a regular basis. Sleep lets the conscious mind rest so the subconscious mind can take over, solve problems, and relieve stress. Sleep brings balance to our lives. Concentration, effectiveness, problem-solving, and energy are all greatly improved when we get enough sleep. Alternatively, all these things suffer severely when we don't. Our patients suffer too. The science and wonder of sleep is amazing. Getting enough of it can often be a challenge.

> When we get enough sleep, our concentration, problem-solving skills, energy, and effectiveness, all greatly improve. Alternatively, all these things suffer severely when we suffer from sleep deprivation.

Although we may commit to getting more sleep, and despite being exhausted, many of us have difficulty falling asleep. Those who work the night shift are at a particular disadvantage. I have always been a night owl, and I loved working the night shift. However, I found that I was eternally tired. No matter how many years we work nights, I think that our internal clocks never fully shift. We cannot fool nature. For those brave nightshifters, sleep is perhaps even more important, and even more elusive. Here are some points to consider as you work towards getting enough sleep.

- **Turn off the television.** TV stimulates our senses. Quiet your mind so you can rest your body.

- **Do something positive.** End your day with something positive – preferably quiet time with breathing, meditation, reviewing your focus items, and physualization. Let go of the day.

- **Stay away from stimulants.** Limit alcohol, caffeine, and/or nicotine several hours before bed. A glass of wine with dinner is fine. Remember that excessive alcohol will cause you to wake in the middle of the night, and you will have difficulty falling back to sleep. The same goes for caffeine and nicotine.

- **Consider a routine.** This can be a challenge for nurses who work varying shifts.

Going to bed at the same time each night (or day) improves your chances of falling asleep. In addition to the same bedtime, it is also useful to have a pre-sleep routine. Things that you could incorporate into your routine include having a soothing cup of herbal tea, breathing, meditating, physualizing, reviewing your focus items, and reaching out to your source. Do a few minutes of yoga or Pilates to stretch and relax. Have a peaceful shower or bath. Listen to soothing music. If you have children, take a few minutes to admire them peacefully sleeping, and kiss them good-night. Do what works for you.

The bottom line is that you need to take time out for yourself – however you do it. Make taking time out a priority. Schedule it into your life. Think of it as part of a care plan for *you.*

Notes

[1]Henry David Thoreau quote retrieved July 28, 2005 from   http://www.brainyquote.com/quotes/quotes/h/henrydavid166869.html

References

Flanagan, Maggie, RN (2005, November). Every Patient Deserves a Safe Nurse (Patient Safety cannot be achieved when nurses are not safe). *AJN, American Journal of Nursing, 105*(11), 12.

Strategy 3

Breathe

"He lives most life who breathes most air."
– Elizabeth Barrett Browning[1]

As nurses, we learn the anatomy, physiology, and chemistry of breathing. But we most often think of breathing only in terms of our patients. Firstly, *are* they breathing? What is the rate, quality, and effort of their breathing? What is their oxygen saturation, and how does their ABG look? We rarely, if ever, **think about our own breathing**. Who has time? *You do.* The fact is that with a simple conscious deep breath, you can relieve stress, clear your thinking, and renew your energy. It is probably the single most important strategy we can use "in the moment" to relieve stress.

Breathing is supposed to be a natural and effortless thing. What we often do not recognize is that, when our bodies and minds are stressed, our breath becomes shallow, which means that less oxygen gets into our bloodstream and, consequently, to our brain. We already know that stress contributes to illness and injury. Neurobiology has taught us recently that, along with elevating our blood pressure, stress physiologically impairs our function. Not only are we physically tense, and likely holding our shoulders to our ears, but our thinking and judgment are impaired. Imagine all the tense bodies, shallow breathing, and impaired thinking going on in nurse's stations all over the world. Now *that* is scary!

Andrew Weil, MD, (cited in Dougherty, 2003) summed it up best when he said, "In just one breath you can begin to change your physiology, your thinking, and your emotional state" (p. 12). When we look at breathing as more than just a natural reflex and consider it consciously, we begin to recognize that the benefits of breathing are wondrous. Therapeutic breathing is simple, relatively easy to learn, and **we can take it with us wherever we go.** In addition, as healthcare workers, we can offer our patients a valuable therapy and a fantastic gift. We can remind them of this natural gift that they already possess and help them fine-tune it.

Patrick Dougherty, a licensed psychologist with 25 years of experience, incorporates Eastern practices such as breathing, visualization, and Chi-Gong into

Western medicine and holds workshops geared towards nurses and psychotherapists. Dougherty offers this insight about the benefits of breathing:

> Beyond stress reduction there are a myriad of ways that teaching breathing and using one's mind can be helpful. Teaching an arthritic client to visualize energy flowing through their arthritic joints as they inhale and visualizing the pain recede as they exhale has been a helpful strategy in the East for centuries. Some patients are very open and wanting to use breath and imagery working with cancer and other chronic illnesses. Even with terminally ill patients, breathing and visualization can ease the pain and help facilitate a smoother transition to death. (2003, p. 2)

Like Mr. Dougherty, many people have discovered and utilized the mind's inherent ability to consciously heal the body.

The mind, body, and spirit are undeniably connected. Eastern philosophies have taught us so much about this connection, as well as specific ways to harness the power of our minds to affect specific changes in our spirits and bodies. I encourage you to explore this fascinating arena in greater detail as you evolve, expand your awareness, and learn to live your life without stress and with your whole soul. For now, I will introduce you to a few key elements of breathing that have helped me tremendously. I am confident that they will work for you too. With minimal effort, you can achieve astonishing results.

- ## Be conscious of your breathing

Begin by being conscious of your breathing. Be aware of the actual mechanics of your breathing. No matter how stressed you are, or how little time you think you have, **with a simple breath you can release tension and negative energy.** I am guessing you are sitting down as you are reading this (unless your life is so chaotic that you cannot sit even for a few moments, in which case, you *really* need this book!). Put your hand on your lower abdomen, *relax* your body, and concentrate on your breathing. Breathe slowly and deeply. Now close your eyes and really *focus.* Feel the air moving in through your nose, filling your lungs and feeding your body, and flowing out through your mouth. Try doing this for two minutes. Chances are, if you are new to therapeutic breathing and conscious relaxation, two minutes will seem like an eternity. Whether you realize it or not, in the past two minutes your shoulders have probably fallen from your ears, your blood pressure has just lowered, and your stress has begun to dissipate.

When things are hairy at work, and you feel you do not have even a moment to get away, remind yourself that you can still release that negative energy and stress. Believe it or not, you can practice this and many other strategies just walking to the bathroom. You know how to get there without thinking about it. On your way, put your hand on your belly (I'd recommend keeping your eyes open) and concentrate on your breathing. Instead of reading the drivel posted in the bathroom, take the opportunity to close your eyes and keep focusing on your breathing. Suddenly, you have turned a quick bathroom break into a stress-releasing revitalizer. It may not be ideal, but sometimes we have to take it where we can get it.

Speaking of all the in-your-face "friendly" reminders and communication in the bathroom *(Can we not get a moment's peace?!)*, why not replace them with something peaceful or something that encourages us to practice our relaxation techniques? Let's face it, those few seconds in that bathroom may very well be the only time we get to ourselves in an entire shift.

The point is this: become conscious of your breathing. Take the opportunity to breathe wherever you are. Whether it is walking to the bathroom, typing on a keyboard, or playing with your kids, remind yourself to really *breathe* throughout the day.

- **Hold Steady**

Another strategy that I love is the Hold Steady. When someone is ranting in the nurse's station, everyone seems to join in. The old mob mentality definitely holds true here. Instead of joining in the bitch-fest, try to *hold steady* with your breathing. Notice how everyone else will reflexively and unconsciously revert to even more shallow breathing as they get more worked up. Take a nice deep breath while holding your peaceful glance steady on the person spouting off negative energy. You will find that she will either let it go and deflate, or she will walk away frustrated to find someone else to suck into her drama. Either way, you win.

• Take Breath Breaks

Taking breath breaks is another useful tool. Periodically throughout the day, stop everything, close your eyes, and simply take 6 to 12 deep conscious breaths – preferably outside. If you can, practice some physualization as well. Although you only need seconds, the more time you give yourself, the better off you will be. It does not take long, and you will recharge in an instant. Give it a shot.

Get creative. Encourage one another to take Breath Breaks. Explore new avenues. Have a signal – either a word or a look – that lets your co-worker know when she is giving off negative energy or when she might need to take a break. Consider posting notes saying *"Breathe"* on the phone or computer screen, so that each time the phone rings or you sit down to the computer, you are reminded to stop and take a therapeutic breath. Consider using the old Pavlovian Response – pick a certain color to indicate and suggest a certain relaxation technique. For instance, you might decide that every time you see the color red, you will take a therapeutic deep breath and consciously release. Before long, you will naturally and automatically breathe, and therefore, *relieve stress* every time you see blood, ambulance sirens, or a stoplight. If it seems too easy, it is.

There is so much to be gained from learning about breathing and the powerful effects of therapeutic breathing. I am only just beginning myself. There are countless books and programs available to assist you as you learn to focus, relax, and energize your body through breathing. Visit the list provided at the end of this book. I would also encourage you to visit www.breathing.com and research Patrick Dougherty's Web site at www.breathingqigong.com to explore some of the options available to you. Dougherty works with nurses and those in health care to utilize therapeutic breathing techniques. Do it for yourself, and do it for your patients. We have so much more to offer our patients when we understand and practice conscious and therapeutic breathing.

Notes

[1]Elizabeth Barrett Browning quote retrieved July 28, 2005 from http://www.aboutbreathing.com/articles/to-all-health-professionals.htm

References

Dougherty, Patrick. (2003). Healthcare and Qigong – Nursing, (p. 2). Retrieved June 13, 2005 from www.breathingqigong.com

Strategy 4

Walk

"My grandmother started walking five miles
a day when she was sixty. She's ninety-
seven now, and we don't know where in
the hell she is." – Ellen DeGeneres[1]

We nurses know a thing or two about walking, don't we? We often feel as if we have run a marathon by the time we finish a shift. Our feet ache, our bodies hurt, and our minds are exhausted. Unfortunately, although there are some health benefits to be gained by the countless steps we may take during a shift (try wearing a pedometer one day to see just how far you travel), those benefits are often outweighed by our poor eating habits, our unhealthy responses to stress, and our lack of exercise when we are not working.

We all know we should exercise regularly and why. The American Heart Association (2005) recommends at least moderate exercise for 30 to 60 minutes most days of the week. Regular exercise has been proven to prevent heart disease and slow or reduce atherosclerosis. It lowers blood pressure, reduces cholesterol, reduces your risk for physical injury (assuming you don't trip and fall on your way out the door), stimulates the lymphatic system, and boosts immunity. It decreases the risk and complications of Type 2 Diabetes, encourages weight loss, and may even help prevent breast cancer in post-menopausal women (perhaps because it helps keep estrogen levels down).

What we might not realize are the wonderful *emotional* effects associated with regular exercise. If you simply get moving, you can actually reduce levels of stress and depression. Those who engage in regular exercise also report an increase in energy and ability to concentrate, along with more confidence, better quality of sleep, and an improved body image.

I remember the first time I experienced the notorious "runner's high." I was a slightly pudgy, very self-conscious teenager vacationing with my family. We were staying in a hotel that happened to have a gym. My younger brother and sister, who were both superstar athletes, were right at home and bounced effortlessly from one piece of equipment to the next. I happened to hop on a treadmill (it looked the least likely to cause embarrassment or bodily harm), and I became hooked. I began exercising regularly and loved what it did for me. Although at that age, I was mostly concerned with what size I could wedge into, the emotional benefits far out-weighed any physical ones. My energy level, self-esteem, and confidence improved. Having once been painfully shy, I began to emerge from my shell, and I began to let the world see who I really was. Looking back, I can see that so much of my personal and emotional growth had to do with just getting my body moving. As I write this, I cannot help but wonder where along my journey I lost that mind-body connection. I am so grateful to have found it again.

On a more scientific note, the American Psychological Association (APA) (2004) tells us that exercise may not cause a rush of endorphins as we once thought. But rather, "One line of research points to the less familiar neuromodulator norepinephrine, which helps the brain deal with stress more efficiently." The APA (2004) article "Exercise Fuels the Brain's Stress Buffers" describes the link between exercise and stress in this way:

> Biologically, exercise seems to give the body a chance to practice dealing with stress. It forces the body's physiological systems, all of which are involved in the stress response, to communicate much more closely than usual. The car-

diovascular system communicates with the renal system, which communicates with the muscular system. And all of these are controlled by the central and sympathetic nervous systems, which also must communicate with each other. This workout of the body's communication system may be the true value of exercise; the more sedentary we get, the less efficient our bodies in responding to stress. (p.1)

In other words, by exercising regularly, we are helping our bodies and minds deal with stress more efficiently.

Treadmills, gyms, and scientific studies aside, the good news is that we do not have to run marathons to achieve the fabulous physical and emotional effects of exercise. **Walking may be the ideal aerobic exercise.** It is easy to do, and it is kind to your joints. Anyone, at any age, at any fitness level can do it. You do not need a gym or any equipment other than a decent pair of shoes. There is no complicated formula to follow, and you can start today.

Even if you have never exercised in your life, you can begin to reap the substantial benefits of regular exercise by simply walking. For those of you who are gym junkies or long-time athletes, good for you. Still, consider walking for its meditative, visualization, and relaxation opportunities.

Walking can provide us with priceless meditative time. Even if you are lucky enough to find time throughout your day to sit quietly and enjoy what we traditionally think of as meditation, walking can be valuable "me" time. Walking brings with it amazing peace and clarity. I have had some of my most creative and life-changing insights while walking. It is a wonderful opportunity to visualize, concentrate on your breathing, and quiet your mind. At the same time, you will be exercising your body and gaining energy you simply wouldn't have otherwise.

Aside from its long-term benefits, walking can be an immediate stress reliever. If you find yourself overwhelmed, stressed out, and exhausted, take some time out and walk. Even for a few minutes. Get away from the stressful environment and go outside if you can. Remember, fresh air does wonders for your mind and body. Focus on your breathing, and quiet your mind. If you cannot get outside or away from the chaos, take the stairs. At least they are quiet. No matter how tired or stressed out I was, I found that bounding up or down the stairs provided a quick pick-me-up when nothing else was possible. Again, we need to take our moments where we can get them.

Again, I will ask you to make a commitment to yourself. Commit to walking as part of living with your whole soul. We already know that the mind and body are connected and do not act independently of one another. Walking not only strengthens your most vital organs and oxygenates every cell in your body; it clears your mind and releases stress.

Unfortunately, the walking (or running) we put in on the job is not going to cut it. No matter how exhausting it may be, our on-the-job walking is generally not consistent and not sustained. Still, for some people, working a 12 to 16 hour shift may constitute your exercise for the day. That is certainly acceptable. Sometimes we just cannot muster anything else. However, the trick is to balance those days with a healthy eating plan, healthy coping strategies, and time out for you. If you continue to work long shifts, plan to walk on the days you are not working.

Begin slowly. Commit to walking just 10 to 15 minutes twice a week if anything more seems too daunting. Something is better than nothing. You can gradually build up to more frequent walks of longer duration. Get outside as much as possible. Focus on *consistency* rather than intensity. I guarantee that if you stick with it, you will wonder how you ever lived without it. The hard part, like anything else, is just getting started.

If you get excited about your newfound stress buster and want to enlist your friends or co-workers, visit InSTEP with NURSES at www.nursingworld. org/anf/step/htm (American Nurses Foundation, 2005). The American Nurses Foundation will help you organize and reach your fitness goals while you raise money to support education and research that promotes public health and advances nursing as a profession. The bottom line is that you must make the commitment and put forth that initial effort to get started.

Make the time and *do it.* You will live longer, better, and happier.

Notes

[1]Ellen DeGeneres quote retrieved July 28, 2005 from http://www.brainyquote.com/quotes/quotes/e/ellendege n131597.html

References

American Heart Association. (2005). Physical Activity and Cardiovascular Health: Questions and Answers (p. 1). Retrieved August 25, 2005 from http://www.americanheart.org/presenter.jhtml?id entifier=830

American Nurses Foundation. (2005). InSTEP with NURSES (p. 1). Retrieved June 20, 2005 from http://www.nursingworld.org/anf/step.htm

American Psychological Association. (2004). Exercise Fuels the Brain's Stress Buffers (p. 1). APA Help Center. Retrieved August 25, 2005 from http://helping.apa.org/articles/pdf.php?id=25

Strategy 5

Let It Go

"Things without remedy, should be without regard; what is done, is done."
– William Shakespeare,[1] *Macbeth*

This chapter introduces you to methods you can use "in the moment" to *let go of* or *release* stress. It is all well and good to lose yourself on the massage table, but it is an entirely different challenge when stressors are firing at you from every angle at work, and there seems to be no escape. Like the rest of the *HealThy Nurse* strategies, these methods are universal and simple, yet surprisingly effective. We cannot eliminate stress from our lives and certainly not from our workplace. However, **we can learn how to manage and release stress effectively and not be held captive by it.** We can learn to stay calm and focused amidst the chaos.

We automatically put up a protective resistance when stressful situations present themselves. We may adopt dysfunctional coping mechanisms and escape mechanisms so we don't have to deal with the bad thoughts and feelings (so we think). We may lash out at a co-worker or, worse, a patient. We may bottle it up until we get home and toss back a few too many drinks or watch that fourth hour of television without even being aware of how we are hurting ourselves.

When we do not face stressful situations or feelings head on and dissolve them, they build up until, as with Selye's stack of paperwork, stress overloads us. The hidden, unresolved pain gets worse, and we become more and more unhappy, burned out, and resistant to our environment. We hold on to and stuff away our bad feelings without even realizing that we are doing it. Before we know it, we are living with exhaustion, fear, stress, and anxiety, and these feelings become so familiar that they are almost comfortable.

As we discussed earlier, true change cannot come without awareness. Most of us react to life unconsciously. So often, reality clashes with our beliefs or the way we think things *should* be. We get so wrapped up in our thoughts, pictures, and stories about the past and the future, and how we think things *should* be, or how other people *should* react, that we miss the simple truth. Some things are out of our control, yes. But *our* world does not just *happen* to us. We control our own thoughts. We have a choice. We can choose to heal and evolve, or we can choose not to heal and to continue down a path of self-destruction.

Remember, even when we decide not to choose, we have still made a choice and we have to live with the consequences. We can choose to live in the moment, knowing that the only time in existence is *now*. **We can choose to become more conscious and less reactive.** We can live our own life, the way we want to live it, with our whole soul.

The stress release methods that we will discuss in this chapter are offered as a starting point. Understanding the importance of relieving or releasing stress on a regular basis and as you move along throughout your day is only one piece of the puzzle. Understanding it means nothing unless you actually *let go* of the bad feelings. As with everything else, you must make the choice, make the commitment, and be persistent.

One of the keys to managing stress is being able to *recognize when you are stressed.* What are your trigger points? Be aware of what gets to you and when you have been gotten to. Then use the following methods, along with the rest of the strategies provided, to escape the stress and burnout that have been holding you back.

1. *Remember that you have a choice*

This may seem redundant and simplistic, but I cannot emphasize enough the power of choice and of realizing that *you own that power.* It does not matter what life or work throws at you – *you can choose how you respond.* You can choose to practice any number of the relaxation or release techniques provided in *HealThy Nurse.* You can choose to reframe your thinking. It only takes a quarter-second.

In their book, *What Happy People Know: How the New Science of Happiness Can Change Your Life for the Better*, authors Dan Baker, PhD, and Cameron Stauth discuss **"the life-changing quarter-second."** Research has shown that there is a quarter-second delay between the brain's urge to take an action and actually taking that action. Baker and Stauth point out that

> This means that every urge you will ever have – including every fearful urge and every angry urge – contains a quarter-second window of opportunity in which you can disengage from that urge. The significance of this is extraordinary. One-quarter of a second may not sound like much time, but in the arena of thought, it's a vir-

tual eternity. It's more than enough time for you to choose to interpret perceptions differently. This quarter-second is your ultimate power over perception. (p. 135)

For instance, say you are overwhelmed at work, short-staffed, and anxious about getting everything done. Instead of thinking to your self, *"I'll never get all of these meds out on time. Will this shift ever end?!"*, reframe or replace those thoughts with positive ones. Say to yourself, *"If I stay relaxed and focused, take it one step at a time, I'll get everything done. I know I'm doing the best that I can."*

So often, we do not even realize how negative and self-defeating our thoughts are. When we are overwhelmed and stressed, we often forget that we have a choice. Remember that *you* control your thoughts. They don't just happen. You will be amazed at what this simple shift in thinking can have on your entire state of mind.

2. *Breathe*

Again, simply breathe. Remember, *with a simple breath you can release tension and relieve stress.* Add a conscious, slow, cleansing breath at the beginning and end of the previous positive scenario, and you are in even better shape. Give yourself cues – for example, pick a color that will remind you to *breathe.* You can wear it or post it around the nurse's station and even in patient rooms.

3. *Stretch*

Each strategy builds on the other. When you recognize that you feel stressed, anxious, or tense, you can choose to focus on your breathing and stretch your body. When we are stressed, we become hunched over and contracted without even realizing it. This can become a chronic state for many of us, and we simply *exist* this way. Stretch your body. If you are sitting, stand up. Slow your breathing, and free your mind. Reach for the sky (metaphorically and literally!), touch your toes, and *breathe.*

4. *Chi Gong*

This body activation / movement therapy is a powerful tool to use "in the moment" to relieve stress and is a great way to literally "shake it off." Stand in a relaxed position, close your eyes, and gently rock and shake your body while focusing on your breathing. Let go of all the negative energy you are holding on to –

feel the negative energy leaving your body (*physualize it leaving your body*). Again, remember to *breathe.* You may need to sneak into the bathroom or break room for this one if you fear your co-workers will dub you a mad woman and get out the soft restraints.

5. *The Sedona Method*®

This technique was developed by Lester Levenson and Hale Dwoskin, who have been practicing and teaching the Sedona Method® since the 1970s. Their books and courses based on this simple, yet transformative practice have helped millions of people. I encourage you to visit Hale Dwoskin's web site at www.sedona.com and Lester Levenson's web site at www.lesterlevenson.org for more information.

The Sedona Method® has been proven to greatly reduce stress, with research showing significant reductions in heart rate, blood pressure, and muscle tension. Dr. Richard Davidson of the State University of New York, a leading researcher in the field of stress reduction, and Dr. David C. McClelland of Harvard University conducted research on the Sedona Method® and praised it "for its simplicity, efficiency, absence of questionable concepts, and rapidity of observable results" (Davidson & McClelland cited in Dwoskin, 2003, pp. 1-3).

The Sedona Method® can be used to reduce stress "in the moment." The method consists of the following 5 steps.

Step 1. **Focus on the fear or anxiety that you are feeling.**

- Be "in the moment" with it and allow it to be, as fully as you can.
- The more you work with this process, the easier it will become for you to identify what it is you are really feeling.

Step 2. **Ask yourself, *"Could I let this feeling go?"***

- This question merely asks you whether or not it is possible to let it go.
- Answer this question with as little thought as possible, and do not second guess yourself (I was famous for second guessing myself – *"I wonder what I'm **supposed** to answer"*).

Let It Go

- Avoid any internal debate about the merits of each answer. *"Yes"* or *"no"* are both acceptable answers, and you will often release or let go even if you answer *"no."*

Step 3. Ask yourself, "Would I?" or in other words, "Am I willing to let go?"

- Again, stay away from the internal debate. It does not matter if your fear or feeling is justified, longstanding, or right or wrong. Follow your gut instinct.
- If you answer *"no,"* or if you are not sure, ask yourself, *"Would I rather hold on to this feeling or be happy and free?"*

Step 4. Ask yourself the simple question, *"When?"*

- This is an invitation to *let it go now.* You may find it easy or difficult to let go.

Step 5. Repeat the preceding four steps as often as needed until you are free of that particular feeling.

Remember that letting go of negative feelings is a decision that you can make any time you choose. If you decide to hold on to a negative feeling, recognize that it is your choice. Ideally, you will find yourself letting go a little more each time, and with a little less effort. Commitment and persistence pay off.

Remember that, as with the other concepts and strategies in *HealThy Nurse*, understanding the importance of letting go a little bit each day means nothing unless you actually do it. With practice and with awareness, you will gradually become less reactive to your environment and more and more able to consciously choose the thoughts, reactions, and feelings you wish to embrace in your life.

All of these strategies work to release stress "in the moment." As with the others, they are offered as a starting point. Figure out what works for you. Once you embrace the concept of letting go and understand why it is a *necessity,* you can create and perfect your own strategies. Be aware that we often become so comfortable with our

> *Remember that letting go of negative feelings is a decision that you can make any time you choose.*
> *If you decide to hold on to a negative feeling, recognize that it is your choice.*

unhealthy coping mechanisms that we may fail to recognize them.

It is easy to blame our unhappiness or our burnout on outside influences. However, as nurses and as human beings, we cannot always control our environment. No one can. The very nature of our work is stressful, and we are bound to be faced with more than we think we can handle from time to time. But you *can* let go of stress no matter how hectic your shift is or how supportive – or unsupportive – your work environment is. These simple tools are effective and beneficial. The implications for nurses who use these tools are wide-reaching. They will make a difference in your life if you decide to use them. **The decision is yours to make.**

Notes

[1]William Shakespeare quote from T. Edwards, C. N. Catrevas, J. Edwards, & R. E. Browns (1959), *The New Dictionary of Thoughts – A Cyclopedia of Thoughts* (p. 468), (no city): Standard Book Company. This quote was also retrieved October 5, 2005 from quoteland.com/1/OpenTopic?q=Y&a=tpc&s=586192041&f=436194441&m=2761938986&p=2-101k– Supplemental

References

Baker, Dan, PhD. & Stauth, Cameron. (2003). *What Happy People Know – How the New Science of Happiness Can Change Your Life for the Better.* New York: Rodale & St. Martin's Press.

Dwoskin, Hale. (2005). The Sedona Method. Scientific Evidence and Results. (pp. 2-3). Retrieved July 16, 2005 from www.sedonamethod.com

Levenson, Lester. (2003). The Release Technique. Retrieved August 28, 2005 from www.lesterlevenson.org

Strategy 6

Activate

"We must always change, renew, rejuvenate ourselves; otherwise we harden."
– Johann von Goethe[1] (1749-1832)

Most of us view a massage as a special treat – something we rarely indulge in. I remember feeling almost guilty as I lay on the table thinking, "I shouldn't be spending money on this. There are a hundred other things that I should be doing. I haven't really earned this." Then I finally realized that activating my body on a regular basis greatly enhances my life. Yes, that massage feels good at the time and in the moment, but we carry so many benefits into the rest of our day, our week, and our life. Body activation, also known as bodywork, includes a general collection of therapies, including massage, body movement and awareness, and energy balancing.

From the beginning, nurses have recognized the therapeutic value of touch – a comforting hand on the shoulder of a frightened patient or a massage to alleviate pain and promote relaxation. As caregivers, we understand that instinctively. Yet, with today's pressures and with time always seeming to elude us, we have regretfully fallen away from that. And we certainly do not consider the benefits of bodywork for ourselves.

Therapeutic Touch was introduced to nursing as a scientifically based process in the early 1970s by Dolores Krieger, RN and Dora Kunz (Nurse Healers, 2005, p. 1). Critics propose that Krieger's findings were based more in religion than in science and that her claims to be able to "read" a patient's energy field were more along the lines of snake oil salesmen of the last century. The whole notion of Therapeutic Touch as paranormal or mystical faith healing is *not* what I am encouraging.

Rather, when we *activate* our bodies – through touch or movement or stretching – a healing energy circulates that is vital to a healthy happy life. Once we begin to nourish and care for our spirit, exploring body activation is a natural progression. We can facilitate our body's own healing response through any number of massage or movement therapies. We can re-charge our bodies and energize our minds and souls. We can ease tension and promote relaxation, reduce pain and soothe injured or sore muscles, as well as stimulate blood and lymphatic circulation. Again, you must choose. Like everything else, incorporating body activation into your life requires a commitment. The different therapies or modalities available are vast. To be honest, I find them dizzying. I invite you to research them for yourself and figure out what works for you. In my mind, body activation is not limited to traditional massage. And energy balances, auras, and mojos may not be up everyone's alley.

You may find that a good facial provides you with the body activation, stimulation, and release from tension that you need – not to mention a healthy glow and a few less blackheads. Remember, all of these strategies are interrelated. Take your meditation where you can get it.

The point is to *do it*. Commit to making it a part of your routine. Do not sell yourself short by making excuses, or by thinking you are not worthy or that you cannot afford it. Many forms of body activation are free of charge, yet valuable beyond measure. For those therapies that do cost money, work it into your budget just as you would your groceries. You must feed your soul too. You absolutely *are* worth it, and the stress and anxiety you leave behind with each session will benefit everyone around you.

If you only do *one* thing, if a once weekly (or even monthly) session on the massage table is all the "me" time you can muster, and you simply cannot make time for the rest of the strategies, then it's a good start. Massage – or any other form of body activation – is a good way to sneak in a little quiet time, a little meditation, a little reflection, and a little breathing, and it is a good way to release the stress and tension you may not even know you are harboring.

This journey toward a healthy mind, body, and soul is all what we make it. If you need permission, take it from me. Your families and patients will thank you. The more we learn about and engage in these healthy alternative therapies, the more we have to offer those around us.

Research has shown that office workers who are massaged regularly perform better and are more alert, and they are less stressed than those who are not massaged (ICBS, 2005). I believe it's safe to assume that most of our patients would prefer that we be more alert and less stressed. Take your own poll. Do your own research.

I find it interesting that we are making such tremendous advances in science and technology, but the quality of care provided does not seem to measure up. Nurses are frustrated because we are stretched too far and unable to provide the care we know we should. Patients and their families have lost faith. But all the science in the world cannot replace the human touch. Perhaps that is why alternative, holistic, or complementary modalities are becoming increasingly integrated into our scope of practice. They often incorporate the "whole" person, and maybe that is what we have been missing.

I know of at least one hospital that offers six free massages per year to every employee. Just the fact that they have an on-sight masseuse is a step in the right direction. By offering these free sessions, the hospital sends its employees the message that they are valued and that their health and well-being are important. This hospital clearly understands the mind-body connection and the importance of activating the body and releasing stress on a regular basis.

Of course, your organization may be leaps and bounds away from offering free massages or even having an on-sight masseuse. But take heart – and take action. Take a course in therapeutic massage (for which nurses may earn CEUs), and share what you learn with your co-workers. The face of nursing must change to a healthier one in order to survive. We have to start somewhere.

I include here a brief introduction to some of the body activation strategies I have explored and find useful. Again, use them as a starting point and find out what works for you. I am not suggesting that all of these will suit you, or that you will necessarily believe in why or how they work, or that they will deliver all that they promise, but consider that they might. We are too quick to pop a pill when we might be better off considering why we are really hurting and how we might better fix it. In the past, if I had a headache, I would take two Excedrin® and chug a Tab®. I discovered later that I was much better off looking at my diet, my stress level, and how I was managing them. Was I utilizing the healthier tools I had learned, such as breathing, meditation, and body activation?

We must utilize our body's inherent ability to heal itself and consider other possibilities. As a nurse, I am both open and skeptical. I believe that it is arrogant to assume that Western medicine is the only way to heal what ails us. As you explore these alternative methods, notice that many, if not all, of these methods combine the different strategies of *HealThy Nurse* – answering your own call light first, expanding your awareness, physualization, breathing, taking time out, and meditation.

Massage Therapies

- *Swedish Massage.* We are most familiar with Swedish massage. This is what most of us encounter at the gym or the spa. Draped in a sheet, you lie unclothed on a padded table while the therapist uses kneading and gliding strokes to loosen your joints and relax your muscles. Sessions range from 30 to 90 minutes and can cost $30 to $90 per hour.

- *Sports Massage (Deep Tissue Massage).* Sports Massage is not just for athletes. This variation can increase your range of motion and speed recovery of injured or sore muscles. Before a workout, Sports Massage can help prevent injury. After a workout, it can reduce soreness and swelling. The therapist often uses more force and direct pressure than in Swedish massage. Prices are similar to Swedish massage.

- **Acupressure and Acupuncture.** This 5,000-year-old practice stems from the Eastern belief that certain points on the body are connected to various organs and life energy by way of channels or "meridians." Acupuncture practitioners believe that the insertion of very fine needles at precise points on the body restores health by unblocking and balancing the flow of energy in the body. Acupressure is most commonly available in the form of the Japanese therapy called Shiatsu. Acupressure does not use needles. The therapist may use her hands, elbows, knees, and feet to apply pressure to certain points on the body to stimulate "chi" or vital energy. Session length and price are similar to Swedish massage.

- **Reflexology.** Also called *zone therapy*, reflexology has been used as a powerful healing therapy in China for thousands of years.

It was introduced to the USA by William Fitzgerald in the 1900s. Similar to acupressure, reflexology uses deep massage on specific "reflex zones" on your feet, hands, and head to relieve tension, ease pain, and improve circulation in corresponding body parts. Sessions range from 30 to 90 minutes, and you can expect to pay $30 to $100 per session.

- **Trigger Point Therapy (Myotherapy).** Therapists who practice trigger point therapy are often osteopaths. Finger pressure is used to release tension in tight muscles resulting from poor posture, trauma, or overuse. It is said to be particularly effective in treating low back pain. This is similar to acupuncture in that certain "trigger points" are believed to cause pain in different areas of the body. Expect to feel soreness in the area for 1 to 2 days afterward. Session length and cost are similar to the other massage therapies.

- **Myofascial Release.** This form of massage seeks to ease the tension of tight fascia, or connective tissue. Proponents claim that stress, trauma, illness, and poor posture can cause your fascia to tighten up and, ultimately, pull bones and muscles out of place. Using mild sustained pressure, the therapist gently stretches and softens the fascia.

This therapy should not be painful, and it may require several sessions before chronic pain is relieved. Myofascial release is helpful in treating headaches, neck and back pain, and recurring sports injuries. Sessions last 30 to 90 minutes and are similar in cost to other massage therapies.

- *Rolfing®*. Also called *Structural Integration*, Rolfing® was developed by biochemist Dr. Ida P. Rolf more than fifty years ago. This holistic system eases chronic pain and stress. You may lie or stand while the practitioner uses deep, sometimes painful pressure to stretch and realign your fascia.

   Rolfing® usually includes a series of ten sessions lasting 60 to 90 minutes. Those who are certified to perform Rolfing® are required to undergo extensive training at the

Rolf Institute® of Structural Integration (Rolf Institute, 2005, p. 1).

- **Rosen Method®.** This method was developed by former physical therapist and health educator Marion Rosen. It utilizes verbal communication and gentle touch to encourage self-awareness and relaxation. Trained to notice subtle changes in breathing and muscle tension, "the practitioner responds with touch and words which allow the client to begin to recognize what has been held down by unconscious muscle tension. As this process unfolds, habitual tension and old patterns may be released, freeing the client to experience more aliveness, new choices in life, and a greater sense of well-being" (Rosen Institute, 2005, p. 2).

Movement Therapies

Movement therapies are aimed at "retraining" your body to move in a healthy way in order to relieve chronic pain and muscular tension. They take into account that the mind, body, and soul are interrelated, and so, incorporate many aspects of meditation and breathing and visualization. Keep in mind that some types of movement may exacerbate arthritis or other joint conditions. *Of course, always check with your doctor before beginning this or any other exercise program.* More importantly though, *listen to your body.*

- **Stretching.** This familiar therapy was introduced in the last chapter and, like many of the strategies, is useful in many regards. Aside from being a wonderful relaxation and release technique, stretching is valuable for its injury prevention and treatment properties. Remember to move slowly, relax, and *breathe.*

- **Yoga.** Quite simply, yoga means *"union".* It utilizes a series of poses and breathing exercises aimed at realizing the unity of our whole being. Yoga is known for its meditative properties, as well as for reducing stress, lowering blood pressure, stimulating the lymphatic system to remove toxins from the body and for slowing the aging process. Anyone can practice yoga in one form or another. Take what you need from yoga. It may simply be a good stretch, or it may be a balanced workout for you. You may find that it is about that divine dance between your body and soul and the living world around you.

- **Pilates.** The Pilates method of physical conditioning was developed by Joseph Pilates beginning in the 1920s. Pilates has recently become popular among celebrities and the rest of us who want bodies like theirs. But dancers (and others in the know) have been using Pilates to stretch and strengthen muscles for decades. Pilates trains the mind to control the body as it focuses on your "core" – strengthening the muscles around your middle. So, it is especially effective in improving overall body strength, posture, and balance. This is particularly valuable if you suffer from lower back pain. Personally, I find that my Winsor Pilates® DVD series does the trick for me. However, there are also some other very good DVDs available, including the Stott Pilates™ series by Moira Merrithew. Pilates studios are becoming ever more common, and you may find working with a personal instructor just right for you. There are also good books available, such as Alycea Ungaro's *Pilates, Body in Motion* and Brooke Siler's *Pilates Body*.

- ***Trager®.*** Developed by physician Milton Trager, MD, this therapy uses simple exercises and rhythmic touch to reduce stress and relieve chronic pain. The belief is that pain and stress can be relieved by retraining the unconscious mind to let go of chronically inflamed or contracted muscles. "Utilizing gentle, non-intrusive, natural movements, The Trager® Approach helps release deep-seated physical and mental patterns and facilitates deep relaxation, increased physical mobility, and mental clarity. These patterns may have developed in response to accidents, illnesses, or any kind of physical or emotional trauma, including the stress of everyday life" (Trager International, 2005, p.

2). Sessions usually last from 60 to 90 minutes.

- **Alexander Technique.** Created by F. M. Alexander, an Australian actor, near the turn of the century, this method of mind-body integration improves balance, posture, and ease of movement. The student becomes aware of everyday movements, and how she may unconsciously be engaging in constricting movements or causing herself pain. The goal is to improve alignment and relieve tension and pain. This technique is often taught at pain clinics and rehab centers. A session may last 45 minutes and cost $35 to $80.

- **Feldenkrais®.** This therapy aims to restore full range of motion to those who have developed inhibited patterns of movement. Without realizing it, we may hold our whole body differently as a result of a sore back or a pulled neck muscle. As a result, we have pain in other areas and set ourselves up for further injuries. The Feldenkrais® practitioner's aim is to guide you through various movements, making you more aware of subtle nuances that can have a major impact on how you move or hold yourself. Look for a properly certified practitioner, and be aware that multiple sessions are recommended.

- **Rebounding.** This zero-impact exercise yields many benefits. It is fun, easy, and safe for almost everyone. It involves simply bouncing on a mini-trampoline in a series of small controlled movements. Rebounding improves circulation, muscle tone, coordination and balance. It increases the capacity of the heart and the lungs. And it reduces stress and increases energy.

- **Swimming.** Swimming allows us to engage in a full range of body activation. Our muscles are relaxed *and* utilized at the same time. The weightlessness takes pressure off our joints and body. Do laps if you want, but play as well. It feels good just to *float and be.*

- *Chi Gong (also Qigong and Chi Kung).* This 5,000-year old Chinese practice is recently gaining popularity in the US. Chi Gong is based on the body's chi (qi) or vital force, and it is related to both tai chi and yoga. Chi Gong fosters self-healing and inner harmony by combining the disciplines of mind, body, and chi. The synchronized breathing and guided visualizations of Chi Gong have many variations. With static or moving Chi Gong, one "shakes" out the blocks of energy (caused by stress and tension) and allows the body's natural chi to flow more freely. It combines breathing, meditation, and visualization. I practice this frequently to relieve stress "in the moment."

In addition to these methods, you may also wish to explore the benefits of aromatherapy, hypnotherapy, and detoxification or cleansing programs. Dance and drumming are also powerful tools that promote relaxation and allow us to let go of stress, especially for those who do not like to be touched. As you explore these forms of body activation, you will become increasingly aware of your body and your mind, and of the connection between them. Body activation will become a way of life for you. However you choose to do it, make the commitment to activate your body on a regular basis to maximize your body / mind / soul connection.

Notes

[1]Johann Wolfgang von Goethe quote from Jeanna Bozell (2003), *A Nurse Leader's Little Instruction Book – The Ultimate Resource for Retaining Staff* (p. 18), Muncie, IN: NurseQuest®, a division of Professional Resource Group, Inc.

References

ICBS, Inc. (2005). Massage Therapy – Benefits of Massage. Retrieved October 20, 2005 from http://www.holistic-online.com/massage/mas_be nefits.htm

Nurse Healers – Professional Associates International. (2005, March 18). TT (Therapeutic Touch) Facts (p. 1). Retrieved July 12, 2005 from http://www. therapeutic-touch.org/newsarticle.php?newsID= 18

Rolf Institute of Structural Integration. (2005). About Rolfing® (p. 1). Retrieved August 28, 2005 from http://www.rolf.org/about/index.html

Rosen Institute. (2005, September). What is Rosen Method® movement? (p. 2). Retrieved August 28, 2005 from www.rosenmethod.org

Siler, Brooke. (2000). *The Pilates Body*. New York: Broadway Books.

Trager® International. (2005). What is the Trager® Approach? (p. 1). Retrieved August 28, 2005 from www.trager.com/approach.html

Ungaro, Alycea. (2002). *Pilates, Body in Motion*. New York: DK Publishing.

More Information

The Alexander Technique
www.alexandertechnique.com

The American Center for fhe Alexander Technique, Inc.
www.acatnyc.org

Chi Gong
www.roaringlionpublishing.com

Feldenkrais® Method
www.feldenkrais.com

Massage Therapy
www.massagetherapy.com

Rolfing®
www.rolf.org

Rosen Method®
www.rosenmethod.org

The Trager Approach
www.trager.com

Pilates
Winsor Pilates®
www.winsorpilates.com

Stott Pilates™
www.stottpilates.com

Strategy 7

Meditate

I am reluctant to use the word *meditation*. To many of us, meditation conjures up images of a bald guy draped in a sheet on top of that proverbial mountain, contemplating the meaning of life without having any grasp of the "real world." I have always been familiar with meditation because my grandmother and my mother practiced it as far back as I can remember. As children, my siblings and I found that my Mom's meditation pyramid, a prop meant to accelerate tranquility and well-being, made a much better fort than a vehicle for inner work.

Quite frankly, no one I knew who practiced meditation seemed to emit the serenity and inner peace it promises. Although I longed for that elusive peace and calm myself, and I had tried meditation throughout my life, I was never able to quiet my mind long enough to get anywhere. I would sit there with my eyes closed, and my mind would race. I would think about what I was thinking about, and what I needed to be thinking about, and where I wanted to go for dinner, and whether the jeans I was wearing made my ass look fat. So, my attempts at meditation were short-lived, and I inevitably drifted away from it. I used to think of meditation as an altered state of consciousness. I now realize that it is just the opposite. Meditation is an *unaltered* state of consciousness.

My journey into meditation was born out of self-preservation rather than anything else. My life was so frantic, and my struggles with work were overwhelming. I began sitting in silence because I had to. It was either that or soft restraints and the psych ward. Without really realizing what I was doing, I learned to meditate.

I would instinctively go someplace quiet; close my eyes, focus on my breathing, and try to let it all go. Sometimes I would have great results and feel energized, peaceful, and relaxed. Other days I would just cry. (*Please* do not discount the healing and de-stressing power of a good cry!) And still other days, it seemed as though my mind would not quiet, and I could not reach any state even resembling relaxation.

Rather than get discouraged by my setbacks, I began to explore meditation more deeply. I learned that this powerful healing tool has been around for thousands of years and is part of every culture – like so many other ancient practices that work in modern life. The world we live in – *especially* the nursing world – is a busy and demanding one. Even if you find the fast pace exciting, you still need to decompress and de-stress on a regular basis. Whether you are an adrenaline junkie or not, nursing is filled with high stress, anxiety, worry, and a workload that never ends. Our minds and bodies can tolerate only so much without becoming saturated and shutting down. We must give ourselves a chance to release the stress and be refreshed on a regular basis.

I prefer to think of meditation as conscious or chosen relaxation. It takes the pressure off. And, to be honest, I don't feel like such a flake. In the end, meditation is simply quieting our minds

> *I used to think of meditation as an altered state of consciousness. I now realize that it is just the opposite. Meditation is an **unaltered** state of consciousness.*

with the ultimate goal of *clearing* our minds of all the clutter. When we sit quietly, close our eyes, and focus on our breathing, it forces our minds away from all the stress and chaos, and it allows us to truly *let go*. It does take discipline and practice, but the results are amazing and worth every effort.

The Science of Meditation

Our brain is continuously generating electrical impulses that rhythmically fluctuate in specific and distinct patterns known as brain wave patterns. The four most commonly known and studied categories of brain wave patterns are Beta, Alpha, Theta, and Delta (a fifth category, Gamma waves, is the most rapid and least studied of the brain wave patterns). Each pattern, measured by an electroencephalography (EEG), correlates closely with our state of mind, our feelings, our thoughts, various body system functions, and even our quality of life.

1. ***Beta Brain Wave Patterns.*** These are the most rapid of the patterns and are found in normal waking consciousness. Beta brain wave patterns are responsible for increased alertness, concentration, and cognition.

This is where our patients hope we function. However, at higher, more rapid levels, Beta brain wave patterns are associated with less desirable conditions, such as angst, panic, and *dis-ease*. Unfortunately, this is the state in which many of us function on a daily basis.

2. **Alpha Brain Wave Patterns.** Brain activity slows to the Alpha wave pattern as we become more relaxed. We are better able to focus, absorb, and recall information quickly when we are in the Alpha state. This state is also known as the "twilight state" between wakefulness and sleep. We might find ourselves in this state when we are absorbed in a good book or as we practice physualization.

3. **Theta Brain Wave Patterns.** Theta waves are slower than Alpha brain waves and are associated with meditation, deep relaxation, and dreaming sleep. Aside from being a state of tremendous stress relief and increasing endorphin production, the Theta

pattern is associated with a number of other beneficial states, including increased insight, creativity, and memory abilities.

4. ***Delta Brain Wave Patterns.*** The slowest of the brain wave patterns, Delta brain waves are associated with deep, dreamless sleep and trances. Although people are generally asleep and thus, unaware while in this state, there is evidence that it is possible to train yourself to remain alert. This state has long been associated with profound healing, deeper meditation, and major boosts in creativity, awareness, and inner peace.

Once we appreciate the impact of our minds on our bodies and, ultimately, on our life experiences and happiness, we begin to understand the importance of quieting our minds. When we meditate, we are consciously slowing our brain waves to achieve a more peaceful and relaxed state. The trick is finding what works for you. It can be difficult to find a few moments alone, never mind allowing or encouraging your body and mind to be still. As with everything else, it takes a

Meditation & the Stress Response

Herbert Benson, MD, associate professor of medicine at Harvard Medical School and president of the Mind/Body Institute at Beth Israel Deaconess Medical Center in Boston, MA, has studied the physiological effects of meditation for over 30 years. He has this to say about meditation.

"Meditation is but one form of relaxation that leads to a common set of physiologic changes.... Physiologically, it is called the relaxation response, and its opposite is the stress response. With the relaxation response there is decreased metabolism, heart rate, blood pressure, rate of breathing, slower brain waves. That's been proven repeatedly in studies." (Benson, cited in Davis, 2000, p. 1)

commitment and a willingness to *make the time* for yourself.

Ideally, we should meditate at least once a day. I find that making it part of my time out, along with phy-sualization and reviewing my focus items helps. Commit to a time that works for you, find a quiet place, sit comfortably, close your eyes, and focus on your breathing. Start there. It's as simple as that. Do some research. Practice different methods. The important thing is that you *do it*. If this is new for you, start small. Give yourself 5 to 10 minutes (it may seem like an eternity at first) and gradually build up to 20 to 30 minutes a day.

Be kind to yourself. Do not expect miracles with a few sessions. Keep at it. And consider what meditation really is for you. Perhaps you get that release, calm, and quiet with a long walk or a bike ride or listening to relaxing music. So you're not in that Delta or even that Theta state? So what! It beats the rapid Beta state of anxiety and chaos in which most of us function. However you do it, explore the possibilities of slowing and quieting your mind on a regular basis. Explore meditation.

What does all this mean in terms of healing and stress?

By meditating, either in the traditional sense or with a peaceful walk, we can help to regulate our brain wave patterns and, thus, the biochemical source of stress, thereby dramatically reducing stress. With a bit of discipline and continued practice, you can experience dramatic improvements in your sense of well-being, self-awareness, ability to learn, focus and concentration, memory, and intuition, as well as enhanced creativity and energy. And you will begin to heal yourself.

The Benefits of Meditation

Meditation has been found to
- *reduce stress*
- *relieve pain*
- *reduce high blood pressure*
- *help unclog arteries to reverse heart disease*
- *increase blood flow to the brain (by helping to reverse arteriosclerosis)*
- *decrease heart rate*
- *decrease respiratory rate*
- *slow brain waves*
- *help relieve PMS, hot flashes, and insomnia*

All of these help to decrease risk for heart attack and stroke. – Davis (2000, p. 1)

Practicing and learning about meditation or conscious relaxation is, of course, beneficial to us as healthcare workers. With this knowledge, we can offer our patients so much in terms of pain relief, an understanding of the importance of the mind-body connection, and a sense of calm and peace that no prescription or pill can bring.

Those who have practiced meditation for years tell us that, eventually, with practice and commitment to a deeper meditative state, our brain reorganizes, and our body reaches a state whereby it can handle all the extra stress and chaos it receives. This means that, by practicing meditation and the other strategies in *HealThy Nurse*, we can become happy and healthy, we can live with our whole soul, and we can be that calm amidst the storm of life. With commitment and continued practice, I intend to discover this for myself.

Notes

[1]Franz Kafka quote from Deepak Chopra (1994), *The Seven Spiritual Laws of Success – A Practical Guide to the Fulfillment of Your Dreams* (p. 20), San Rafael, CA: Amber-Allen Publishing & New World Library.

References

Davis, Jeanie Lerche. (2000, May). The Mysterious 'Medication' of Meditation (p. 1). WebMD Medical News. Retrieved 11/05/05 from http://www.webmd.com/content/Article/25/1728_57992.htm

More Information

Learning meditation
(This site provides a "meditation room" with auditory programs to guide you through various meditative sessions as well as a suggested reading resource. This Web site is free.)
www.learningmeditation.com

Hope for the Future

"When spider webs unite,
they can tie up a lion."
– Ethiopian Proverb[1]

Most of us love our profession, but we are disenchanted, and we are feeling the painful effects of burnout. The good news is that, despite feeling frustrated and exhausted, we still have a burning desire (or at least a flickering desire) to help others and to make a difference in the nursing profession.

In her book *Where Have All The Nurses Gone?*, Faye Satterly, RN writes,

> The shortage is a problem that isn't going away. It has taken more than a decade and a variety of factors to create and will require more than just the efforts of hospital administrators to resolve. It will require assistance from physicians and support from the public, and some of the issues will need to be addressed by the nursing profession itself, particularly the overwhelming reticence of its members to communicate to others the value of their work. (p. 14)

I believe that **the only way the nursing industry can be transformed, and a potential catastrophe in**

healthcare averted, is by changing the industry one nurse at a time. We can all take back our lives and our careers, and we can look toward a happier future. The principles and strategies provided in this book are simple and have been proven over centuries to be powerful and beneficial. They worked for me and they can work for you.

> *"There is mounting evidence that unhealthy work environments contribute to medical errors, ineffective delivery of care, and conflict and stress among health professionals. Negative, demoralizing and unsafe conditions in workplaces cannot be allowed to continue. The creation of healthy work environments is imperative to ensure patient safety, enhance staff recruitment and retention, and maintain an organization's financial viability."* – American Association of Critical-Care Nurses (2005, p. 4)

Improving the Work Environment

When I left my position in the Emergency Department I met with my manager to turn in my resignation, and I was a bit surprised by the response I got – a very flip *"OK!"* and a curt smile. After all those weekends, holidays, coming in on short notice, and long hours, I couldn't help but wonder where the *"Sorry to see you go."* or *"Is there anything I can do?"* was. After all, I was a first-rate employee by all accounts. I had always received excellent annual reviews and was never "called into the office" or disciplined. I got along well with the staff, and I had an outstanding attendance record. I could not believe that I had brooded over my decision to leave and that I worried about "letting my team down" by walking away. In the end, it was clear to me that I was completely disposable and that loyalty meant nothing. My experience left me wondering why any of us stay.

Throughout my research, I learned that feelings of being disposable and undervalued are common among nurses. I remember a time when my co-workers, including the doctors, were like family, and we felt a very real sense of commitment. The truth is that the strongest bonds that keep nurses satisfied with their jobs are their relationships with co-workers and, in particular, managers.

Nurses have spoken out in countless surveys and studies, such as the landmark national survey of RNs in the United States conducted by *NurseWeek* and the American Organization of Nurse Executives (Graham, 2002). While money absolutely does matter, recognition, respect, support, and *less stress* are crucial to both retention and recovery. Many RNs report that they plan to leave their present job and the profession within the next few years. (This is not surprising. Haven't we all experienced the negative impact the nursing shortage has had on patient care?) Many nurses would not recommend their place of employment to a loved one, and even more would not recommend nursing as a profession. We're seeing a greater number of patients per nurse and a higher turnover among experienced RNs.

These staffing problems are part of the vicious cycle that nurses are trapped in, and is the direct result of burnout. We will all need a nurse one day – whether it's *your* mother, *your* child, *your* husband, *you.* What kind of care will *you* receive?

There is much talk about recruitment these days. It seems so simple to me. It can cost up to 1.5 times an RN's annual salary to recruit and train a new nurse (Capponi, 2005, p. 12). It is an expensive and lengthy process. Keep in mind that this new nurse is statistically not likely to remain in her position for more than a year or two. To put this in perspective, if retention plans save just 15 positions, hospitals would save over a million dollars per year in retention money. If 25 positions are saved through retention, *hospitals could save nearly 2 million dollars in one year* (p. 12).

Hospital executives and recruitment campaigns are focusing on marketing and advertising. Much of retention and recovery, on the other hand, is minimal in cost. Remember that there are a half million trained and licensed nurses who are not currently practicing (Department of Health & Human Services, 2002, p. 2) as a direct result of poor management, long hours with few breaks, high stress, and burnout. Thousands more say that they plan to leave the profession in the near future. So, recruiting new nurses is certainly part of the solution, but if we do not fix what is broken, the new nurses won't be far behind those choosing not to use their degrees.

It is true that nurses must take responsibility for their own happiness and job satisfaction. However, management can do a great deal to nurture nurses and make nursing a healthier profession to be part of. As nurses, we need encouragement, mentoring, and coaching so that we, in turn, can do the same for each other. Moreover, we need to work to change the attitudes that prevent us from working together as a team. I believe that beating stress and burnout and that living a healthy, happy, whole-souled life will take us a long way towards reaching these goals.

The results of the extensive on-line survey done by the American Nurses Association revealed that of the nurses who plan on leaving their jobs, many say they would consider staying if certain conditions were met. Chief among these conditions are better compensation, improved work environment (including more resources and less stress), better hours, and more respect from management (Graham, 2002). Money is tight. We all know that. But three of the four biggies on their wish list require only some creativity and a willingness to try something different. This study found that although "money is important," "other factors, including job stress and professional status may

> **The principles and strategies provided in this book will work for everyone.**
> *If our leaders are healthy and happy, they will lead by example. If managers encourage their nurses to live the principles and strategies in HealThy Nurse, we can all make a difference and help transform our ailing industry.*

be even more critical" (Graham, 2002, p. 3). Neither of these things have to cost a thing. Additionally, the survey found that of those nurses who have left the profession, almost half said that a less stressful work environment would likely cause them to consider returning.

In order to work towards increased retention, we must strive to make our troubled work environments as positive as possible. Managers are leaders, and retention is all about leadership. Many nurse managers earn their promotions as a result of their outstanding clinical skills (even though they may have little management experience or training). But it seems that after trading in their scrubs for street clothes, they quickly forget what it's really like "in the trenches." Nurses often feel as though management makes important decisions dictating nursing practice based solely on bottom-line numbers and without having any idea what it takes to give excellent, or even adequate, patient care. However, if we can work together to give nurses more authority to make decisions about scheduling, staffing, policies and procedures, and allow them to exercise their critical thinking skills, every nurse will feel empowered and will give better care at the bedside.

Unfortunately, many of those in leadership positions are struggling with burnout themselves. Organizations need to focus on more leadership training and on providing managers with the real-life powerful tools that are needed to deal with the stresses of their position, so that they can be better coaches for their staff. **The**

principles and strategies provided in this book will work for everyone. If our leaders are healthy and happy, they will lead by example. If managers encourage their nurses to live the principles and strategies in *HealThy Nurse*, we *can* make a difference and help transform our ailing industry.

We all must work to improve relations with hospital leadership. Mutual respect is key. We must get away from the suits and scrubs mentality. If we are asking for respect, we must give it. And we must *be* the professionals we know we are. As with the Boomerang Principle, we must be willing to accept what we ask for. Nurses must be willing to take action, make decisions, and be accountable for those decisions.

Towards achieving this goal, I urge you to get involved. Familiarize yourself with legislation such as the Quality Nursing Care Act, which

> builds on more than a decade of research showing that RNs make the quality difference in patient care and that when RN care is insufficient, patient safety is compromised and the risk of death is increased. The proposed legislation mandates the development of staffing systems that require the input of direct-care RNs, and it provides whistle-blower protections for RNs who speak out about patient care issues, including

inadequate levels of nurse staffing. (Indiana State Nurses Association, 2005, p. 1)

The nursing profession desperately needs legislation like the Quality Nursing Care Act in every state, and in every country.

In addition, we need legislation to ensure adequate school funding. In December 2004, the National League of Nursing (NLN) reported that 125,000 nursing school applicants are turned away each year as a result of a critical shortage of teaching faculty. Increased funding is needed to accommodate the increased enrollment that is resulting from recruitment campaigns such as "Discover Nursing," sponsored by Johnson & Johnson, and "Agenda for the Future," sponsored by the American Nurses Association. Because of the requisite low student-to-teacher ratios in nursing schools, costs are much higher than in other departments. During the last serious nursing shortage in 1974, the federal government allocated $153 million for nurse education programs. In today's dollars, that would be $592 million – nearly *four times* what congress is currently spending. It leads one to wonder whether our federal government takes the looming shortage seriously (Bonalumi, 2005, p. 18).

> *There are solutions to the many problems facing the nursing profession today.*
> *I challenge every nurse to recognize, understand, take responsibility for, and conquer her own burnout.*
> *Focus on progress, not perfection. It will not happen overnight, but it will happen.*
> *Just knowing that you are taking positive steps and doing something about it can put a new and positive spin on your life. By beating burnout, you can do your part to heal nursing.*

Aside from the American Nurses Association (ANA), which we are all familiar with, there are a great many nursing organizations that support and empower nurses. What is, perhaps, most important is getting involved in your own hospital, office, or organization. Lead by example. Start a trend. Engage others. Encourage them to take breaks, use healthy strategies to relieve stress, and answer their own call light first. We all know that our patients need to be more accountable for their own health. **We too need to be more accountable for our own health**.

Although it would be ideal for your co-workers and your nurse manager to become as enthusiastic about *HealThy Nurse* as you, the beauty of choosing this new life is that it doesn't matter if they come along for the ride or not. Remember, you can't change others. You can only change yourself.

As for managers and administrators, give us a reason to stay! I am not, nor have I ever been, a manager. But after working with no less than five different managers in ten years, I know bad management. The feeling that loyalty doesn't matter echoes among nurses these days. And it's no wonder, considering how many of us watch fellow nurses hop from one sign-on bonus to the next, staying only as long as their contracts require. Those of us who are dedicated and stick it out through the tough times are forced to wonder why. Why are those of us who have been loyal and who have "paid our dues" forced to work the same number of weekends and holidays as those new employees? Where are *our* bonuses? Where is the incentive for us to stay?

With all the focus on patient satisfaction these days, we need to redirect some of that energy toward employee satisfaction. After all, you cannot have one without the other. Nurses need to know that those long hours, weekends and holidays away from our families, and that bad back are all worth it. Quite simply, nurses want recognition.

Speaking of recognition, let's talk money. Looking back, nurses have not seen a significant increase in salary since the nursing shortage of the 1980s (Bradley, 2002, p. 1; Satterly, 2004, p. 112). That's nearly *two decades!* Meanwhile, workload, responsibility, and risk for personal injury have increased exponentially and continue to climb. It is astonishing that many organizations still do not increase nurses' pay for demonstrated competence and/or certification in a specialty field. These nurses, incidentally, are known to be at higher risk for burnout.

Yes, nurses are altruistic, but we do not come without a price. With our salaries not budging for decades when adjusted for inflation, we can't help but feel as if our employers are taking our loyalty for granted. A coupon for a free ice cream cone ("recognition" where I worked) is both unprofessional and insulting. In her book *Where Have All The Nurses Gone?*, Faye Satterly, RN points out that

> While money is not the strongest draw for nurses, the implication of appreciation and value that is attached to wages is. Even in times of cost containment, there has to be some salary recognition for nurses to compete with other areas of employment. (p. 112)

The bottom line is that **money talks, and it does matter.**

Redefining Nursing

Improving the work environment is one aspect of resolving the shortage and beating burnout. *Redefining nursing* is another, perhaps equally daunting, piece of the puzzle. If we do not want history to continue repeating itself, we must work to advance nursing as a profession. Through the years, I have at times felt both proud and a little embarrassed to say that I am a nurse. While nurses are seen as caring, trustworthy, and altruistic, most people still harbor huge misconceptions about what nursing really is.

When asked, many people mistakenly associate nursing with crisp white hats, bedpans, and menial tasks. We are seen as laborers. If nursing is viewed as little more than a dead-end vocational job, why on earth would bright, innovative, and driven young people be drawn to it? Recruiters speaking to high school students about nursing typically hear that many view nursing as both stressful and scary, with terrible hours and little chance of advancement (Domrose, 2002). Hmmm, this is all true. *What the hell was I thinking?!* We have to get the message out there that nursing can also be an extremely rewarding and exciting profession. When recruiting prospective students, we need to make it clear that our field is science-based and not the red-headed stepchild of healthcare.

According to *NurseWeek* (2002), Americans love nurses but have a narrow view about what we really do.
- *Only half of Americans know that RNs must have a bachelor's or an associate's degree.*
- *Fewer than one in five know that nurses must be licensed.*
- *Less than 20 percent of Americans know that RNs must have continual education.*
- *More than two in three Americans do not know that nurse practitioners are allowed to prescribe drugs."*
(statistics from the Johnson & Johnson study cited in Domrose, 2002, p. 3)

That said, when luring prospective students into nursing, recruiters and recruitment campaigns tend to avoid sharing the somewhat unpleasant realities about how tough the job really is. We need to be honest about what nurses will face when they get out of school, and we need to provide them with the tools to deal with the stress and ugliness they will encounter. Otherwise, they will quickly burnout and abandon the profession like so many others. New nurses joining the workforce hardly stand a chance if the nurses orienting or mentoring them are burned out, cynical, and negative about their profession. Therefore, money spent on recruitment efforts will be wasted unless more energy is devoted to retaining and satisfying the nurses we already have.

Acceptance of nurses as professionals is not only hampered by the public's misconceptions, but by nurses as well. My friend and fellow nurse, Barb, has always said that nurses could be such a powerful force if we could just quit bickering and stop acting like a bunch of school girls. Obviously, most nurses are women. (According to The Center for Nursing Advocacy, 2005, only 5% of nurses are men. I apologize to those few brave men for the female pronouns throughout this book.) I was excited to see the headline "Nurses Discuss Recent Changes in the Field" in my local newspaper (Louvar, 2005). I was, however, disappointed to find it in the "She" section in the back, right next to the article "Denim Moves Uptown" and a recipe for Peach Ambrosia.

Quite frankly, it's no wonder that more men don't get involved in nursing, and that, if they do, they don't stick around. The nurse's station can feel like a junior high cafeteria with all the gossip and catfights. If we want to be treated like professionals, then we must act like professionals. Period. I believe that most of the bickering and complaining comes from pain. When we are over-stressed, tired, and don't know how to effectively cope and relieve the pain, we take it out on others. However, when we realize that we have the choice to replace our ineffective coping mechanisms with other healthier behaviors, we can immediately change the atmosphere in that nurse's station.

As we work towards improving our image as professionals, keep in mind that nurses lose credibility when we are overweight, reek of cigarette smoke, or otherwise emit an unhealthy image. Although we frequently joked in the Emergency Department that stupidity is job security, the truth is that most people are not stupid. Our patients recognize the contradiction.

Degree requirements in nursing have been hotly debated recently. In order for nurses to be seen as professionals, educational requirements should become more uniform. As it stands now, the knowledge and skill level of a "nurse" can vary tremendously with little distinction in our practice. I believe that making a bachelor's degree mandatory for all future entry-level nurses is essential in order to earn the respect we desire and deserve in our profession. A study published by the Journal of the American Medical Association (JAMA) in September 2003 found that raising the percentage of RNs with bachelor's degrees from 20 percent to 60 percent would save four lives for every 1,000 patients undergoing routine surgeries (Aiken, Clarke, Cheung, Sloane, & Silber, 2003).

Obviously, I am not suggesting that we make all current nurses who do not hold a bachelor's degree go back to school. There *is* a critical shortage after all. Before I go any further, let me say that I feel honored to have had an LPN as a mentor and friend. Carolyn was one of the best nurses I have ever had the pleasure of working with. Sometimes no amount of education can replace years of experience and good instincts. However, with almost daily advances in science and technology, nursing is becoming increasingly complex. In order to be viewed as professionals, we must set higher minimum requirements for those entering the field. Requiring a bachelor's degree for new nurses must be considered.

Another unpopular thought is that, along with recruitment and retention, we must also consider weeding out the "bad" (*gasp!*) nurses. We all know nurses – hopefully you don't know many – who absolutely scare us. I have come across nurses who can barely form a proper sentence, have zero common sense, or just simply shouldn't be nurses. We wonder how they sneaked through high school, never mind nursing school.

I am not for a second suggesting that we let nurses go without good reason, but perhaps we should be less lenient for the sake of simply having another warm body on the unit. I propose that many of the "difficult" nurses didn't start out that way. Maybe they are burned out and need help. The *HealThy Nurse* principles and strategies may be just what they need.

The relationship between nurses and doctors has been fodder for many a scandal over the years. We've all heard horror stories of doctors screaming at nurses and degrading them in front of anyone within earshot. I like to think it happens less frequently, but it is obviously still socially acceptable, as evidenced by its continued practice. In a 2002 survey for the American Journal of Nursing, almost 90 percent of respondents *"had witnessed yelling, public berating of nurses by doctors, and abusive language"* (Rosenstein, 2002, cited in Satterly, 2004). Although we talk of an interdisciplinary team approach to health care, it doesn't always *feel* that way. The condescension can be palpable. Doctors must take heed and realize that their ability to practice will suffer if nurses continue to burnout and the nursing shortage goes unchecked.

In their defense, doctors are feeling the effects of burnout too. Many of them are overwhelmed and struggling in a field that has changed tremendously over the years – seemingly not in their favor. Like us, they have

> *"In the hospital, the gap between the 'doers' (the doctors and nurses) and the 'thinkers' (administrators) is unbridgeable. We are responsible for actual patient care, and they are responsible for their own asses. When we are in the trenches, they are in meetings. The really don't have a clue."* – David L. Gregory,[2] MD, FACEP, 30 year ED Physician

watched "patients" turn into "customers" who want instant gratification and a quick fix *("Do you want fries with that?")* without taking any responsibility for their own health. If doctors and nurses can finally work towards a *truly* collaborative relationship built around mutual respect, we can then tackle our struggling healthcare field together. We'll all be much happier, and our patients will most definitely receive better care.

There *are* solutions to the many problems facing the nursing profession today. I challenge every nurse to recognize, understand, take responsibility for, and conquer her own burnout. Focus on progress, not perfection. It will not happen overnight, but it *will* happen. Just knowing that you are taking positive steps and doing something about it can put a new and *positive* spin on your life. By beating burnout, you can do your part to heal nursing.

I implore nurse managers and those in leadership positions to think outside the box and consider alternatives to what is **clearly not working.** Remember that when you are stressed, your staff is stressed. Decreased employee satisfaction leads to decreased patient satisfaction. That's a bottom line that any manager or administrator can understand. Recognize that **the number one reason nurses leave their position or the profession is their relationship with their manager or immediate supervisor.**

Thankfully, there are nurses out there who are leading the way and working to change the nursing profession. Sharon Cochran,[3] MSN, RN talked with me about her work as the retention coordinator for Clarian Health Partners at Riley Hospital for Children in Indianapolis, Indiana. She is refreshingly passionate about her job and about nursing. Her excitement resonates as she talks about her work. In the four years since beginning the retention program, she has seen the turnover rate drop from **17% to 2%.** She has witnessed a dramatic increase in nurse satisfaction, and states that burnout and stress within her organization are not as prevalent as they were even one year ago. She reports that there are currently zero staff nurse vacancies in her hospital and waiting lists on some units.

Sharon Cochran attributes the increase in job satisfaction to a number of factors, among them, the hospital attaining Magnet status and living up to all that it implies, a career advancement program, and a Healing Healthcare program. Although she is the retention coordinator for the entire hospital, she says that "The unit manager is the chief retention

I implore nurse managers and those in leadership positions to think outside of the box and consider alternatives to what is _clearly not working._
Remember that when you are stressed, your staff is stressed. Decreased employee satisfaction leads to decreased patient satisfaction. Recognize that the number one reason nurses leave their position or the profession is their relationship with their manager or immediate supervisor.

person. She is the most important person in terms of her staff satisfaction."

Sharon points out that what is so often missing is the relationship between nurses and management and helping nurses recognize their contribution. She says,

> Nurses want to feel like they are appreciated and recognized. And **it needs to be authentic** – not just a pat on the back. The type of praise is important. Tokens, happy retreats, and team building fall short. They are treating the symptom and not the problem. It's dismissing them for who they really are.

She says that authentic recognition means that nurses are included in decision-making and recognized for the experts they are. It means that nurses feel like someone is really listening to them and really cares about them as whole human beings.

Exit interviews, a common measure used to determine employee satisfaction, are "too late" according to Sharon. Instead, she does both intention and satisfaction interviews, as well as periodic focus groups. She told me, "I'm into prevention." Despite working under unusually stressful circumstances, she often hears even seasoned nurses declare, *"I love my job!"*

As nurses in her organization begin to *feel* that authentic appreciation and as they take more accountability for their own behavior, Sharon sees them get excited about their practice again as they recognize that they make a difference. She reports a distinct shift "from the influential people being the complainers to the influential people being the positive, enthusiastic ones." And she says, "Give me an angry nurse. That means they still care. There's a lot of energy in that anger and it can be turned into excitement and enthusiasm. I always say that I sing to the choir and add to the choir one at a time."

Sharon Cochran is a wonderful example of how those in management positions can use innovative measures to make a difference and help heal nursing. Likewise, *HealThy Nurse* offers nurse managers just such an opportunity to affect change and make a difference. Managers, I encourage you to practice the principles and strategies we've discussed here, and to encourage your staff to practice them. Lead by example.

Try introducing your staff to a new strategy every week, and then follow up to see how it's working for them. Get creative. Consider introducing your staff to new ways to relieve stress. Many hospitals are incorporating integrated or alternative medicine into their repertoire. Why not invite someone from another department to talk to your staff about the powerful effects of therapeutic massage or other ways to reduce stress? Be supportive. Ask for feedback and *listen.* Nurses see right through that transparent "smile and nod" so familiar among nurse managers. We know when we are really being heard and when we're not. Explore new avenues to relieve stress and rejuvenate the mind. Get excited and share that excitement with your staff. Help them get passionate about nursing again. You'll find that it is contagious.

Nursing is a job we take with us wherever we go. For all the stress and drama, I cannot imagine a more rewarding profession. Nursing offers so much – science, healing, flexibility, the ability and opportunity to help save lives. The rewards are *immeasurable.*

It is easy to loose sight of that when we become so stressed and unhappy. *HealThy Nurse* can help you overcome stress and escape burnout. It has the potential to help you change your life. But that can only happen if you make the decision to allow it to do so. By taking personal responsibility for our own happiness, remembering the seven basic principles, and practicing the seven basic strategies, we can eradicate the root cause of burnout and, as a result, eliminate the epidemic nursing shortage – *one nurse at a time.*

Notes

[1]Ethiopian proverb quote retrieved February 18, 2005 from http://www.worldofquotes.com/proverb/Ethiopian/1

[2]David L Gregory, MD, FACEP, in personal communication October 12, 2005.

[3]Sharon Cochran, MSN, RN, in personal communication September 12, 2005.

References

Aiken, L. H., Clarke, S. P., Cheung, R. B., Sloane, D. M., Silber, J. H. (2003). Educational levels of hospital nurses and surgical patient mortality [Electronic version]. *JAMA, Journal of the American Medical Association, 290,* 1617-1623. Retrieved July 28, 2005, from www.jama.com

American Association of Critical-Care Nurses (AACN). (2005). *AACN Standards for Establishing and Sustaining Healthy Work Environments – a Journey to Excellence.* Retrieved October 20, 2005 from http://www.aacn.org/aacn/pubpd

cy.nsf/files/HWEStandards/$file/WHEStandards.
pdf

Bonalumi, Nancy. (2005, September). Nursing Faculty: the other side of the nursing shortage. *ENA Connection (The Official Newsletter of the Emergency Nurses Association) 29*(7), p. 18.

Bradley, Carol. (2002, April 8). Taking the plunge (p. 1). *NurseWeek*. Retrieved February 18, 2005 from http://www.nurseweek.com/ednote/02/040802_print.html

Capponi, Nanci. (2005, April). Nurse Recruitment Versus Nurse Retention: A Different Perspective. *ENA Connection (The Official Newsletter of the Emergency Nurses Association) 29*(3), p. 12.

Center for Nursing Advocacy. (2005). How many nurses are there? and other facts (p. 1). Retrieved February 2, 2005 from http://www.nursingadvocacy.org/cgi-bin/print_article.cgi?article_url=http://www.nursinged

Department of Health and Human Services, Health Resources and Services Administration, Bureau of Health Professions, National Center for Health Workforce Analysis. (2002). *Projected Supply, Demand, and Shortages of Registered Nurses: 2000-2020*. Retrieved July 28, 2005 from ftw://ftp.hrsa.gov/bhpr/nationalcenter/rnproject.pdf

Domrose, Cathryn. (2002, June). Mending our image – Americans love nurses, but the public still has a narrow view about what the profession actually does. New media campaigns try to polish those perceptions and draw potential RNs into the fold (p. 3). *NurseWeek.* Retrieved February 18, 2005 from http://www.nurseweek.com/news/features/02-06/image_print.html

Graham, Tim. (2002, April 8). What nurses say (p. 3). *NurseWeek.* Retrieved February 18, 2005 from http://www.nurseweek.com/news/features/02-04/aone_print.html

Indiana State Nurses Association (ISNA). (2005, May, June, July). Nurse staffing bill introduced in US House of Representatives. In *ISNA Bulletin (The Official Publication of the Indiana State Nurses Association) 31*(3), p. 1.

Louvar, Abbie. (2005, May 11). Patient care-providers nurses discuss recent changes in the field (p. C1). *The Republic*, Columbus, IN.

National League of Nursing. (2004, December). News Release. Retrieved August 28, 2005 from http://www.nln.org/newsrelease/datarelease05.pdf

Satterly, Faye. (2004). *Where Have All The Nurses Gone? The Impact of the Nursing Shortage on American Healthcare.* Amherst, NY: Prometheus Books.

HealThy Nurse
Suggested Readings & Resources

Baker, Dan, PhD & Stauth, Cameron. (2003). *What Happy People Know: How the New Science of Happiness Can Change Your Life for the Better.* New York: St. Martin's Press.

Beck, Charlotte Joko. (1989). *Everyday Zen: Love & Work.* San Francisco: Harper.

Benner, Patricia. (1998). *Expertise in Nursing Practice: Caring, Clinical Judgment and Ethics.* New York: Springer Publishing.

Bozell, Jeanna, RN, CPC. (2003). *The Nurse Leader's Little Instruction Book: The Ultimate Resource for Retaining Staff.* Muncie, IN: NurseQuest®.

Cass, Hyla, MD. & Holford, Patrick. (2002). *Natural Highs.* New York: Avery Publishing.

Chodron, Pema. (2002). *When Things Fall Apart: Heart Advice for Difficult Times.* Boston, MA: Shambhala.

Desikachar, T. K. V. (1999). *The Heart of Yoga: Developing a Personal Practice* (rev. ed.). Rochester, VT: Inner Traditions.

Desmond, Lisa. (2004). *Baby Buddhas: A Guide for Teaching Meditation to Children.* Kansas City, MO: Andrews McMeel Publishing.

Fontana, David, PhD. (1999). *Learn to Meditate: A Practical Guide to Self-Discovery and Fulfillment.* San Francisco: Chronicle Books.

Fontana, David & Slack, Ingrid. (2002). *Teaching Meditation to Children: A Practical Guide to the Use and Benefits of Meditation Techniques.* New York: Harper Collins.

Farhi, Donna. (2000). *Yoga Mind, Body & Spirit: A Return to Wholeness.* New York: Holt.

Hendricks, Gay, PhD. (1995). *Conscious Breathing: Breathwork for Health, Stress Release, and Personal Mastery.* New York: Bantam Books.

Institute of Medicine (Corporate Author). (2004). *Keeping Patients Safe: Transforming the Work Environment of Nurses.* Washington, DC. National Academies Press.

Kabat-Zinn, Jon, PhD. (1995). *Wherever You Go, There You Are: Mindfulness Meditation in Everyday Life.* New York: Hyperion.

Kabat-Zinn, Jon, PhD. (1990). *Full Catastrophe Living: Using the Wisdom of Your Body and Mind to Face Stress, Pain, and Illness.* New York: Delta.

Katie, Byron & Mitchell, Stephen. (2002). *Loving What Is: Four questions that can change your life.* New York: Random House.

Korn, Errol R. & Johnson, Karen. (2005). *Visualization: The Uses of Imagery in the Health Professions.* Goshen, VA: EIH Publishing Company.

Levey, Michelle & Levey, Joel. (1999). *Simple Meditation and Relaxation*. Berkeley, CA: Conari Press.

Lewis, Dennis. (1996). *The Tao of Natural Breathing: For Health, Well-Being and Inner Growth*. San Francisco: Mountain Wind Publishing.

Lipton, Bruce H., PhD. (2005). *The Biology of Belief: Unleashing The Power Of Consciousness, Matter And Miracles*. Santa Rosa, CA: Elite.

Luby, Thia. (1998). *Children's Book of Yoga: Games & Exercises Mimic Plants and Animals and Objects*. Santa Fe, NM: Clear Light Publishing.

Maslow, Abraham H. (1987). *Motivation and Personality* (3rd ed.). New York: Harper Collins Publishers.

Monaghan, Patricia & Viereck, Eleanor G. (1999). *Meditation – The Complete Guide*. Novato, CA: New World Library.

Moore, Thomas. (2001). *Original Self: Living with Paradox and Originality*. New York: Harper Perennial.

Moran, Beth, RN, C.N.P. & Schultz, Kathy. (1998). *Intuitive Healing: A Woman's Guide to Finding the Healer Within*. Boston, MA: Houghton Mifflin.

Moyers, Bill. (1995). *Healing the Mind*. Boston, MA: Main Street Books.

Osho. (1996). *Meditation: The First and Last Freedom* (1st ed.). New York: St. Martin's Press.

Plummer, George W., MD. (2003). *Consciously Creating Circumstances.* Whitefish, MT: Kessinger.

Rechtschaffen, Stephan, MD. (1997). *Timeshifting: Creating More Time To Enjoy Your Life.* New York: Doubleday.

St. James, Elaine. (1995). *Inner Simplicity: 100 Ways to Regain Peace and Nourish Your Souls.* New York: Hyperion.

Satterly, Faye, RN (2004). *Where have all the Nurses Gone? The Impact of the Nursing Shortage on American Healthcare.* Amherst, NY: Prometheus Books.

Selye, Hans, MD, PhD. (1978). *The Stress of Life: The famous classic – completely revised, expanded, and updated with new research findings* (2nd ed.). New York: McGraw-Hill.

Siler, Brooke. (2000). *The Pilates Body.* New York: Broadway Books.

Stevens, Bobbie R., PhD. (2001). *Unlimited Futures: How to Understand the Life You Have and Create the Life You Want.* Naples, FL: Tara Publishing.

Tolle, Eckhart. (2004). *Power of Now: A Guide to Spiritual Enlightenment.* Novato, CA: New World Library.

Ungaro, Alycea. (2002). *Pilates, Body in Motion.* New York: DK Publishing.

Weil, Andrew, MD. (1998). *Health and Healing: A look at medical practices – from herbal remedies to biotechnology – and what they tell us.* New York: Houghton Mifflin.

Wenig, Marsha. (2003). *YogaKids: Educating the Whole Child Through Yoga.* New York: Stewart, Tabori and Chang.

Wilson-Schaef, Anne. (2004). *Meditations for Women Who Do Too Much* (rev. ed.). New York: Harper Collins.

Nursing Web sites

American Nurses Association
www.nursingworld.org

Bureau of Health Professions
www.bhpr.hrsa.gov

Nurses for a Healthier Tomorrow
www.nursesource.org

Sigma Theta Tau International – Honor Society of Nursing
www.nursingsociety.org

Web sites related to *HealThy Nurse*

Breathe
www.breathingqigong.com
www.breathing.com

Let Go
www.sedona.com
www.lesterlevenson.org

Activate
www.rosenmethod.org
www.trager.com
www.massagetherapy.com
www.winsorpilates.com
www.stottpilates.com
www.rolf.org
www.alexandertechnique.com
www.acatnyc.org (The American Center For The Alexander Technique, Inc.)
www.roaringlionpublishing.com (Chi gong)

Meditate
www.learningmeditation.com